Home Births

Home Births

The report of the 1994
confidential enquiry by
the National Birthday Trust Fund

Edited by

Geoffrey Chamberlain
Emeritus Professor in Obstetrics and Gynaecology
University of London
London, UK
and
Consultant Obstetrician
Singleton Hospital
Swansea, UK

Ann Wraight
Research Midwife
National Birthday Trust
London, UK

Patricia Crowley
Consultant Obstetrician
Coombe Lying-in Hospital
Dublin, Ireland

The Parthenon Publishing Group
International Publishers in Medicine, Science & Technology

NEW YORK   LONDON

The publishers thank R.J. Demarest for permission to use the illustration on the cover of this book, taken from *An Illustrated Guide to Human Reproduction & Fertility Control*, by R.J. Demarest and R. Charon, published by the Parthenon Publishing Group, 1996

Published in the UK by
The Parthenon Publishing Group Limited
Casterton Hall, Carnforth
Lancs. LA6 2LA, UK

Published in the USA by
The Parthenon Publishing Group Inc.
One Blue Hill Plaza
PO Box 1564, Pearl River
New York 10965, USA

British Library Cataloguing in Publication Data
Home births : the report of the 1994 confidential enquiry by the
   National Birthday Trust Fund
   1. Childbirth at home
   I. Chamberlain, Geoffrey   II. Wraight, Ann   III. Crowley, Patricia
   IV. National Birthday Trust Fund
   618.4

ISBN 1-85070-934-3

Typeset by Martin Lister Publishing Services, Carnforth, UK
Printed and bound by Butler & Tanner Ltd., Frome and London, UK

Contents

List of contributors

Geoffrey Chamberlain MD, FRCS, FRCOG, FACOG
Emeritus Professor of Obstetrics and Gynaecology at the
  University of London
Consultant Obstetrician, Singleton Hospital
Swansea SA2 8QA
Wales

Patricia Crowley MB, BCh, DCh, FRSPI, MRCOG, BAO
Consultant Obstetrician
Coombe Lying-in Hospital
Dublin 8
Ireland

Jane Henderson BSc, MSc
Researcher in Health Economics
National Perinatal Epidemiology Unit
Oxford OX2 6HE

Miranda Mugford BA, DPhil
Economist
National Perinatal Epidemiology Unit
Oxford OX2 6HE

Ann Oakley MA, PhD
Professor of Sociology and Social Policy
Director of Social Sciences
Research Unit
Institute of Education at the University of London
London WC1 0NS

Ann Wraight SRN, SCN, MDD, PGCEA
Research Midwife
National Birthday Trust
London NW1 4RG

Foreword –
1994 Home Births Study

Some of the most profound experiences of my life have taken place at home births. When I was 8 years old my mother had her fourth child at home. Seeing my sister, Sue, so new, so red and smelling so special had a profound effect on me and decided my future career as a midwife. My three beautiful children were born at home and we were exceedingly fortunate in having a very kind and committed midwife for our first birth. She taught me what a difference a midwife can make to the woman's experience of birth. During my career as a midwife I have been at many home births, supporting women and helping them through the pain and the long hours and it seems to me that there are several factors about home births that are important.

Home births allow women more choice. A woman who books for a birth in hospital can only have her baby in hospital; a woman who books for a home birth has doubled her choices, for while she probably will have a home birth, she may end up in hospital because the labour was taking too long, because the pain was too great to be acceptable or because a complication occurred. The woman has much greater control in her own surroundings. She is the pivotal figure around whom the whole world evolves. She can eat and drink what she likes. She can move, groan, moan and take up those positions which make the experience more comfortable. She is assured of privacy – no one can enter her home without her permission. She is in charge – the Boss.

I am deeply honoured and very pleased to write the foreword for the 1994 Home Birth Study carried out by Professor Geoffrey Chamberlain,

Midwife Ann Wraight, and Doctor Patricia Crowley. This informative and comprehensive study of births intended to take place at home in 1994, shows that women who are choosing home births are taking wise decisions, that planned birth at home is a safe option, that the women who are being selected for home births are appropriate and that midwives manage home births well and competently. Professor Geoffrey Chamberlain and his team have done womankind a service by producing these data; he has done this so many times before in many previous studies, all performed so that women can be informed of the safest and most appropriate ways for them to give birth.

Women and midwives are grateful to The National Birthday Trust and this energetic and dedicated team, for throwing light on a controversial subject, debated passionately by many.

Caroline Flint
President, Royal College of Midwives
1996

Preface

The National Birthday Trust Fund (NBTF) having been associated with the active care of mothers and babies before World War II, later turned its attention to surveys of the maternity services. Previous to the Home Births 1994 Study, surveys were conducted in 1946, 1958, 1970, 1984 and 1990 (see Table 1).

Table 1 Previous national surveys on maternity services performed by the National Birthday Trust Fund

	Survey year	No. of births examined	Titles of reports	Publication dates
Maternity in Great Britain	1946	14 000	Maternity in Great Britain	1948
Perinatal Maternity Survey	1958	17 000	Perinatal Mortality	1963
			Perinatal Morbidity	1969
British Births 1970	1970	17 000	British Births 1970 Vol. 1	1975
			British Births 1970 Vol. 2	1978
Facilities at the place of birth	1984	8000	Birthplace	1989
Analgesia in labour	1990	9000	Pain and its Relief in Childbirth	1993

The first of these surveys was conducted by Professor J.W.B. Douglas in conjunction with the Population Investigation Committee. It examined 14 000 births in 1 week of March 1946, the results being published in *Maternity in Great Britain* in 1948. This survey was performed just before the start of the National Health Service and examined the effects of child bearing on the economics of the household. Only a few medical aspects were examined, but details about the relief of pain and method of delivery were analysed.

In 1958, the National Birthday Trust Fund, in conjunction with The Royal College of Obstetricians and Gynaecologists, performed the Perinatal Mortality Survey. Organized by Professor Neville Butler and Professor Dennis Bonham both of University College Hospital in London, it analysed data from 17 000 births in 1 week from England, Wales and Scotland from a very detailed questionnaire completed by midwives. A unique feature of this survey was that for a further 3 months after the clinical survey week, all babies who suffered a perinatal death had an autopsy examination organized by Professor Albert Claireaux, then of Great Ormond Street Hospital. Hence detailed and organized results of the pathology of 7000 autopsies could be correlated with the clinical material. These were reported in two volumes, *Perinatal Mortality* (1963) and *Perinatal Morbidity* (1969).

In 1970 The British Birth Survey was performed by Doctors Roma Chamberlain and Geoffrey Chamberlain again under the joint auspices of The National Birthday Trust Fund and The Royal College of Obstetricians and Gynaecologists. This study investigated the quality of life of the mother and baby in pregnancy and for the first week after delivery with information collected from Scotland, Wales, Northern Ireland and England. It concentrated purposely on the living, dealing with health and morbidity of mother and child, since the 1958 study had examined mortality. Analyses were presented in *British Births 1970, Volume I* (1975) and *Volume II* (1978).

From these national studies three cohorts of children were generated whose antenatal and intrapartum details had been well documented. These are still being followed up by scientific groups, the eldest subjects being almost 50 years of age. Valuable information is still being extracted and published about the development of the children in relation to childbirth and their subsequent life.

In 1980 the National Birthday Trust Fund was considering performing another national survey into obstetrical matters along the lines of the previous studies. By now, however, groups of social scientists and obstetricians round the world were also active in this field. In those days, there was a possibility that the statutory collection of information was about to be expanded by the then Office of Populations, Censuses and Surveys (OPCS). Much of the information which had been collected by the special efforts of the Birthday Trust surveys would then become available from officially collected data sources on a regular and recurrent basis. The OPCS plans never materialized but we were not to know that then. The National Birthday Trust Fund was, in addition, advised then that the collection of cohorts of children in the manner used previously was not necessarily the best way of generating such longitudinal studies. The group of children assembled might be biased in some seasonal way and so could influence the follow-up of education developmental practice. In consequence the Birthday Trust decided not to hold another cohort survey but instead to concentrate on studies in special areas of maternity care.

After 2 years of planning, in 1984 data were collected nationally of staffing and equipment available to women in all the sites of delivery in the country over four separate days in August, September, October and November. This survey was funded jointly by the Department of Health and Social Security and The National Birthday Trust Fund. It was performed by Professor Geoffrey Chamberlain and Miss Phillipa Gunn, a midwife of the National Birthday Trust Fund. Much is published about the expected plans for organization of staff and equipment with proposed levels laid down by the Health Authorities. The National Birthday Trust Fund set out to determine in some detail what was actually happening at the place of delivery. The results were published in *Birthplace* (1987); these were used by health planners as a blueprint for much of the work in the maternity services in the late 1980s in the UK.

The next specialist study was performed in 1990 on the availability and usefulness of pain relief in labour in the whole UK. This was funded jointly by the Department of Health and The National Birthday Trust Fund and was performed by Professor Geoffrey Chamberlain and Mrs Ann Wraight, a National Birthday Trust Fund midwife, with Professor Philip Steer then of the Department of Obstetrics and Gynaecology, Charing Cross Hospital. The use of both pharmacological and non-pharmacological analgesia in childbirth was examined and the opinions of women, their partners and their midwives were obtained allowing a correlation of the birth from three points of view. The results were published in *Pain and its Relief in Childbirth* (1993) and were helpful for the planning of pain relief at a time when women's perception of childbirth and the professionals' management was in a state of formative flux.

All these five surveys have been performed with funds from The National Birthday Trust Fund helped in the past by Government and Royal College funds. The Trust is now combined with Wellbeing, the research funding body associated with The Royal College of Obstetricians and Gynaecologists and it is hoped that the Trust's interests will still go on with other studies in the future that will examine aspects of the care of women and their babies, for that was one of the original aims of the National Birthday Trust Fund in 1929[1].

THE CURRENT STUDY

The survey team comprised Professor Geoffrey Chamberlain and Dr Patricia Crowley (obstetricians at St George's Hospital, London and The Coombe Women's Hospital, Dublin respectively) and Ann Wraight (a National Birthday Trust Fund midwife). It was financed entirely by the Trust and, for the first time, without a contribution from the Department of Health. St George's Hospital Trust and Medical School is thanked for the accommodation offered to the survey team throughout the study. Dr Janet Peacock, medical statistician, and Richard Hulkhory, computer programmer of that medical school, assisted the project team with data analysis and the merging of data sets.

The majority of this report has been completed by the survey team but valuable help was given in specialist areas by Miranda Mugford and Jane Henderson (economist and researcher respectively at the National Perinatal Epidemiology Unit, Oxford) and Professor Ann Oakley (Director of the Social Science Research Unit at the Institute of Education in London) resulting in chapters, respectively, on the economics of home births and the follow-up survey.

Sarah Reed, who was the project secretary and assistant to the midwife director, typed and retyped the script and did much more in the analysis of data; Anne Fraser correlated the many comments written by the mothers, their partners and their midwives.

This study could not have taken place without the women and their midwives who completed and returned the questionnaires. The National Birthday Trust Fund is also indebted to all the Supervisors of Midwives who faithfully co-ordinated the data collection within their own localities; Dr Tricia Murphy-Black and Katherine Pinkerton co-ordinated the Scottish collection.

Many groups and individuals assisted the team:

(1)   Members of the *NBTF Scientific Committee*;

(2)   Members of the *Home Births Study Steering Group*;

(3)   Midwives and Jo Garcia (social scientist) at the *National Perinatal Epidemiology Unit* in Oxford;

(4)   Midwives at the *James Paget Hospital* in Norfolk and *St George's Hospital* in London who took part in the pilot studies;

(5)   The *Stillbirth and Neonatal Death Society (SANDS)* who advised on the questionnaire design for mothers whose babies had died;

(6)   All the *Local Research Ethics Committees* who examined and approved the proposed project;

(7)   Dr Rona Campbell, Dr Charis Glazener, Dr Gavin Young and Dr Luke Zander who shared their knowledge and experience of surveys in examining maternity services;

(8)   Duncan Larkin, the artist who produced the helpful figures;

(9)   The publishers, Parthenon Publishing, who have produced an admirable report.

The Trust has always endeavoured to provide non-governmental data, unopinionated by any one professional group. The information reported in this survey is so presented. Some comments are made by the researchers of the survey from their professional expertise and it is hoped the balance of the editorial team together with the guest authors has provided an equipoise in this highly charged area of maternity care in the UK.

REFERENCE

1.   Williams, S. (1997). *Women and Childbirth in the Twentieth Century. A History of the National Birthday Trust Fund 1928–1993.* (Stroud: Sutton's)

1

History of home birth

ANCIENT HISTORY

Many humans settled in homesteads when they stopped being hunter gatherers in the period 15 000 to 10 000 BC. After the cave period came the building of wattle mud huts. Probably the first organized dwellings were in Mesopotamia, north-east Africa and then the Nile valley. Home was the centre of life where everything happened including childbirth which took place where everyone lived in the common single room. This was the universal pattern.

Not a lot is known about births in ancient history; the better recorded evidence is from the papyri and tomb decorations of Egypt. In ancient Egypt delivery did not occur in the birth house attached to some temples as a few Victorian archaeologists deduced. These were the side chapels for the gods and were not used for giving birth by ordinary mortals, who used their own homes.

In the home, pharmacological pain relief was virtually unknown; although opium and alcohol were used in other aspects of life, most pain relief seemed to be by distraction therapy. Birth was a communal event and when labour started many of the female relatives and women of the village arrived, shrieking in sympathy with the woman in labour.

For a few of the upper classes, a birth assistant may have been at hand to help. She was someone who had attended several births before and so had a little experience. She might bring with her a birth stool, a primitive piece of furniture which has evolved very little to the functional birth chair we have today. The seat was hollowed out in front with two pulling pillars fixed on the arms. The assistant usually sat in front of the stool and made no attempt to intrude upon labour. If the woman was too poor to afford a birth stool she often squatted on two bricks with the perineum off the ground or lent forward on all fours. These positions seemed instinctive and are still seen in many births in Europe today. In this study we report the frequency of their use in the UK still in 1994.

Returning to ancient Egypt; once the baby had been born, the woman was usually carried to her bed. Separation of the baby by cutting the umbilical cord had a religious significance; the ritual of being born was equated with that of rebirth, i.e. entering heaven after death. The umbilical cord was divided with a *pff*, a fishtail-shaped knife. The placenta also had particular religious significance and was usually buried under the hearth of the main room of the house or hut. It was considered to be an important factor for future fertility and so was placed in the threshold where the woman stepped over it frequently[1].

The only clustering of people into institutions in those days probably took place in the temples where people came for conjoined religious worship. There were no hospitals as such but a lot of primitive operations were performed in the home. There were no obstetricians. Although women consulted Egyptian doctors before 3200 BC for a variety of gynae-cological problems, pregnancy and childbirth were just another part of life. Any advice to the woman would be from her relatives or the local village good woman. Should a problem occur in pregnancy or childbirth, a midwife might have been called if there was one available. Doctors were not consulted for they had no idea about obstetrical complications so there was little point in asking for their help.

EARLY CHRISTIAN DAYS

The home still remained the central pivot of society. The Christian Church took over from the organized religions of Egypt, Mesopotamia and Rome but the Christians had to disperse their religious meetings until Christianity became more acceptable in the second and third centuries. Probably the law, the armed forces and entertainment in that order were the next social events that brought people into communal buildings but none of these was associated with health care at childbirth.

MIDDLE AGES

Hospitals came late as collective centres of human health care, existing in this country from the thirteenth century, St Bartholomew's Hospital in

Smithfield being one of the oldest. They mostly looked after the poor, the dying and those who had suffered accidents. Birth was considered a natural event and so took place in the home. Even the advent of doctors as accoucheurs in the seventeenth century did not alter the place of birth.

EIGHTEENTH CENTURY

In 1752 William Smelley, a popular man-midwife, gives an excellent account of births at home of which he attended many[2]. He described how the woman could be seated on a stool made from a semicircle of wood but Smelley considered that the most convenient position for natural and easy labour was:

> ...with the woman lying on the bed upon one side, the knees being contracted to the belly and a pillow put between them to keep them asunder.

He describes how:

> large sheets should be doubled four times, one end being slipped in below her breech while the other end hangs over the side of the couch to be spread on the knee of the accoucheur or midwife who sits behind on a low seat.

As soon as the woman has delivered the baby and placenta, the sheet was removed and a soft warm cloth applied and she was dressed with a clean warm half shift, a linen skirt and a bedgown. Smelley makes passing reference to the Parisian method where the patient half sits and half lies to make the brim of the pelvis horizontal, commenting:

> I consider this is for labours lingering or tedious.

THE START OF THE MATERNITY HOSPITALS

At about the time Smelley was writing this, the first maternity hospitals started in western Europe. In the middle of the eighteenth century, groups of philanthropically minded people realized that the sort of deliveries that Smelley described were satisfactory in the surroundings of the middle and upper classes but not the dirty, crowded and ill-lit homes of the poor, the lower classes and the unmarried. In consequence Maternity and Lying-in hospitals were started, not for medical reasons but for those of charity. In London four were founded within a few years. The General Lying-in

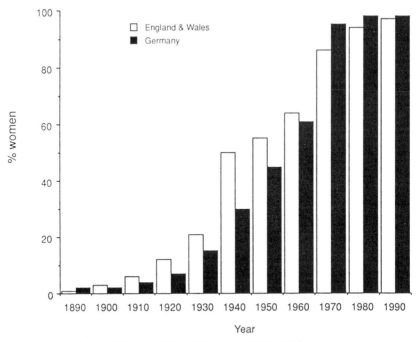

Figure 1.1 Institutional births in UK and Germany, 1890–1990

Hospital, now Queen Charlotte's Hospital for Women, opened in 1748, The British Lying-in Hospital which became the Hospital for Mothers and Babies in Woolwich, in 1749. Sadly this is now closed. The City of London Lying-in Hospital, started in 1750, has now gone too as has the New Westminster Lying-in Hospital founded in 1765. The only London general hospital that had a lying-in ward in the 1750s was the Middlesex where care was shared between midwives and the man-midwife in-ordinary and a man-midwife extra-ordinary, the titles referring to their duties in the hospital or the district. In Dublin the Rotunda Hospital had been established in 1745, in Edinburgh lying-in wards were established in 1756 and the Lying-in Hospital itself established in 1784.

Up to this time, Europeans had always been ahead of the British in maternity matters. Their books were used in translations in Britain and it was not until the 1740s that British obstetricians started to catch up. Many centres of Europe, such as Berlin and Paris, were used by British obstetricians for training and there were maternity hospitals in the major towns of both Germany and France. They were not, however, places where women went willingly. In the middle of the sixteenth century Ambroise Paré was a great teacher at the Hôtel Dieu in Paris. Although deliveries took place here, it was probably not a hospital in the contemporary sense of the term, more a teaching centre where the poor were gathered in order that Paré could teach midwives.

It was not until the end of the nineteenth century that hospitals started to become more widely used in Europe when, for example, in Paris in 1890 there were some 30 000 births occurring at home and 60 000 in public assistance institutions. In Britain, home remained the place for delivery for most of the nineteenth century despite the increase in the number of hospitals. By the turn of the century about 1% of women were having babies in institutions and the rest at home.

THE MOVEMENT FROM HOME TO HOSPITAL

The shift to hospital is basically a twentieth century phenomenon in all countries of the Western World except Holland. It started slowly until after the First World War, since when it has increased steadily. The figures for Britain and Germany are shown in Figure 1.1. They represent the changes in both these Western European countries and would reflect changes in the rest of Europe.

The reasons for this move of women to the institutions to give birth are many. It followed the urbanization of society when people moved from the countryside into the towns. Whilst the industrial revolution took place a century before, farming and agricultural industry had still played a large part in the affairs of the UK and Germany until after the First World War. Thence it declined and the young people moved into the towns where the surroundings in their new homes were often less salubrious than they had been in the country; small apartments and flats were the norm for the young but these were not quite as roomy and pleasant for childbirth as had been the houses they had left. The systems of payment for health changed in Germany in the 1920s and in Britain in the 1940s (the National Health Service, NHS) to allow hospitals to be a more accessible financial alternative for women and this too played its part in the shift.

Perhaps a more important factor was that women now wanted more treatment if emergencies arose in childbirth. They no longer accepted pregnancies that ended badly as Acts of God. From the latter days of the nineteenth century, the middle class began to limit their families by mechanical female contraception with the diaphragm and cervical cap. A stillbirth now became a calamity rather than a blessing as it used to be; women wanted to do the best to get a good result from their pregnancies. The mean family size reduced very sharply around this time and women considered their maternity care to be better in hospital and perceived the hospital to be a safer place to have a baby. This was part of a general drift away from the community into the white-coated environment that happened in most branches of medicine in the 1920s. Hence, while in the nineteenth century the hospital was for deliveries for the poor, the destitute and the unwed, gradually over the next 50 years, the middle classes moved towards institutional delivery.

Did the doctors recommend and enhance this movement? Since most of the specialists and general practitioners were doing their obstetrics outside the hospitals in the first 20 years of this century, it is unlikely that they would encourage hospital births for that would mean losing custom from their paying practices. No doubt as time moved on into the 1930s, the consultant obstetrical staff joined in the movement of women in seeking hospital delivery, but they were by no means the leaders at the beginning of this trend for most of them worked outside the hospital. The benefits of institutional delivery that were eventually considered by doctors were related to the availability of emergency services should they be required. This need might not have been frequent but in the hospital were the equipment, assistance and another doctor to give the anaesthetic.

The position of the British College of Obstetricians and Gynaecologists (BCOG) was interesting. Fletcher Shaw in the early 1930s wrote to Lord Athlone that:

> It should be clearly understood the reduction of maternal mortality would not be secured by increasing the hospital provision for normal cases, but as far as the bare information goes there does not appear to be any reduction in maternal mortality in districts where the larger proportion of mothers having babies is in hospital.

In 1935 a BCOG committee considered the relative places of hospital and home deliveries from a slightly different angle.

> Adequate provision could only be made at great expense because overcrowding in maternity hospitals could cause great peril. It was safer to keep hospital admissions strictly for abnormal accommodation and meanwhile improve domiciliary service until the increase of hospital beds adequate to meet the need is secured.

The financial aspects of the problem were stressed again but there is a hint in the last words that the domiciliary maternity service was not a permanently structured one. The following year the British College prepared a document on aspects of obstetrics *Essential to an Effective*

National Maternity Service[3]. In a section on domiciliary compared with hospital management of labour they stated:

> Women more and more seek hospital accommodation during labour. Hospital provision is essential, chiefly in cases of abnormality or suspected abnormality, but the more successful the ante-natal supervision, the fewer will be the cases requiring transference to hospital after labour has begun. Adequate hospital provision for all cases could only be made at great expense; the results of domiciliary midwifery do not warrant such expenditure.

The same year, the British Medical Association wrote:

> In this respect it is important to note that all available evidence demonstrates that normal confinements, and those which show only minor departures from the normal, can be more safely conducted at home than in hospital. The supervision of maternity as a whole must obviously be conducted almost always under domiciliary conditions.[4]

Some doctors in the mid-1930s said they would be happy to be away from the domiciliary environment which was often squalid. There they were under pressure from well-meaning but unthinking relatives who wanted a prolonged labour brought to a close swiftly. Aiding this trend but for a different reason were some midwives who thought the hospital was a better place. Alice Gregory who headed the British Hospital for Mothers and Babies in Woolwich earlier in the century was pleased to have deliveries at that institution to provide training for her midwives.

Figure 1.1 shows how after the 1920s the increase in institutional deliveries, the converse of home deliveries, increased in almost a straight line so that by the 1980s they made up 95% of deliveries. The decline in home deliveries probably owes more to fashion rather than to any strong medical or midwifery direction. Professionals followed the trend rather than led it. Retrospectively, the professionals tried to justify this move on medical grounds. Similarly, prodomiciliary delivery groups attacked the obstetricians for a trend that had already happened. All this led to confrontations which hardened attitudes on both sides but the debate came too late to stop the already existing trend.

ANALGESIA IN HOME BIRTHS

In the 1920s, only women who were private patients with their own obstetricians had access to pharmacological pain relief. One of the founding resolutions of the National Birthday Trust Fund (NBTF) was to enhance the availability of pain relief for all women. In consequence, the Trust set up a committee with the BCOG in 1933 to investigate the use of analgesics in labour[5]. Four different methods were to be examined:

(1) Nitrous oxide and air from an inhaler;
(2) Chloroform capsules;
(3) Chloroform from an inhaler; and
(4) Paraldehyde per rectum.

After taking evidence, the joint committee considered that paraldehyde per rectum could not be recommended because it did not provide adequate analgesia. It was further concluded that chloroform was not safe to be used by midwives acting alone. This reduced the use of these methods of analgesia in the domiciliary scene. Nitrous oxide was found to be:

> a safe and satisfactory method of analgesia, although the apparatus was expensive and nitrous oxide costly.

The joint committee recommended that midwives should be trained specially in the use of nitrous oxide and women should be medically examined in the last weeks of pregnancy to see if they were fit for 'gas and air'. A great advance came with the production of a light portable machine developed by Dr Minnitt of Liverpool with funds from the NBTF. This cost about ten guineas in the mid-1930s while the British Oxygen Company arranged for the supply, delivery and connection of gas cylinders in the home at a flat rate of 3/6d (17.5 pence). Nitrous oxide was still well used at the time of the 1994 survey by 50% of women at home and 72% in hospital.

Pethidine came to the UK after the Second World War. The Germans had speeded its development as a means of self-administered pain relief for their front line troops and we inherited it from them. Unfortunately, for the first few years of its use, the addictive powers of pethidine were not recognized so some used it for regularly recurrent pains like dysmenorrhoea and became habituées of its use. Such a risk need not be considered for women in labour who only have one or two doses in response to severe pain and for whom there is no danger of addiction. The portable nature of pethidine made it very popular in the 1950s and 1960s, but many women disliked its removal of the sense of control; that, and occasional neonatal respiratory depression, led to a reduction in its use. This is reflected in the report of the current survey when 4% of women at home and 30% delivering in hospital were reported to use it in labour.

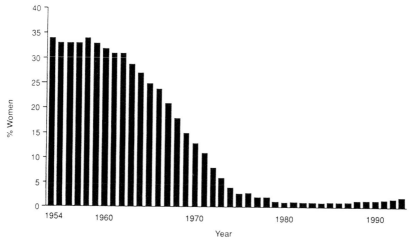

Figure 1.2 Percentage of maternities at home, England and Wales 1954–93 (Office of Populations, Censuses and Surveys)

Epidural analgesia, although started in the 1960s, only became more widely available in the 1980s in the UK. The principal limiting factor has been the number of skilled anaesthetists available to give it. There are still not enough and the general use of epidurals is only common in large hospitals. In the 1994 survey 12% of women delivering in hospital had an epidural or spinal analgesia but obviously none at home.

MORE IMMEDIATE EVENTS

The continued atrophy of the domiciliary midwifery service went on with the various reorganizations of the NHS (particularly that in 1974) and shortly after this the then Department of Health and Social Security proposed a reduction in the maternity services as a whole because of the falling birth-rate. District Health Authority treasurers thought they had found ways of saving money by restricting what was left of a domiciliary service which by then was managing about 10% of births. This was the last straw and home births came down to less than 1% in the 1980s (see Figure 1.2).

During the Second World War the Royal College of Obstetricians and Gynaecologists published a report on a national maternity service[6]. In it they said:

> At the present time there is a shortage and a bad distribution of maternity beds for all classes of the community. There is an urgent

need for the provision of more beds everywhere. From available figures it would seem wise to make provision to begin with for about 70% of all births. The number required for a region giving 15 000 births a year may be reckoned by allowing 20 patients a year for each lying-in bed, with a proportion of antenatal beds equal to one-third of the lying-in beds. For 70% of 15 000 births, on this basis, 525 lying-in beds would be needed and 175 antenatal beds, a total of 700 maternity beds to be apportioned amongst the various maternity centres. The numbers would have to be worked out area by area, the needs of town and country being different.

No evidence is given in the report of why 70% is advised and it seems the first time that this magic figure appears; it is about 20% more than the reported institutional deliveries at that time (51%). This over-provision may have been induced to get a uniform national increase because of the irregular distribution of beds, and so cover the worst areas. This may be an example of using the principle of always asking for more than you need in order to get enough.

The Cranbrook committee, set up by the Minister of Health to produce an official government report[7], repeated this percentage again with no statistical justification:

> ...sufficient hospital maternity beds to allow for a national average of 70% of all confinements that take place in hospital should be adequate to meet the needs of all women in whose case the balance of advantage appeared to favour confinement in hospital.

At that time institutional deliveries made up about 54%. The Association for the Improvement of Maternity Services started in 1960 when home deliveries were about 34%. One of the Association's first objectives was a provision of more hospital beds for maternity services – a reflection of the contemporary anxieties. Hospitals were being mostly used by women for delivery and when in 1970 the Peel report[8] came out institutional delivery rates were already 85%. In this report Sir John recommended:

> We think that sufficient facilities should be provided to allow for 100% hospital delivery. The greatest safety in hospital confinement for mother and child justifies this objective.

This was a recommended change but it must be remembered that the Peel committee was a sub-committee of the Standing Maternity and Midwifery Committee of the Central Hospital Services Committee. It was thus not a ministerial committee as was Cranbrook.

Much has been made of these recommendations as driving forces, directing women into hospital. This is probably not true as the movement had already happened to a large extent. What they were recommending was the provision of facilities for those who wanted to go into hospital. If any driving took place it was the closing down of the domiciliary service through lack of their take-up due to the local management of maternity services rather than any central recommendations of influential obstetricians, general practitioners, Royal Colleges, or Departments of Health.

Much has been made of the safety issue; there are those who would show that the hospital was no safer than a good domiciliary service, for example Tew[9]. While this is patently untrue for all the abnormal pregnancies and deliveries, it may well be true for well-selected women at low risk who have good domiciliary facilities. Unfortunately much of the debate about safety has not distinguished the booked from unbooked or emergency home deliveries. This we do in this study.

In 1974 the Society for the Support of Home Deliveries was set up. In 1986, by which time the proportion of home deliveries in the UK was around 1%, the Society produced a report calling for increased choice in childbirth. They pointed out that home births were about a selection process not a medical problem. This was an important reminder that not all the problems of childbirth are medical but relate to the woman's own attitudes around the time of birth.

The overemphasis on safety was reinforced in the comments made by the Royal College of Midwives in 1987[10]:

> There is some doubt about the assumption that the safest place of delivery for all women is the consultant unit.

A change in emphasis from purely safety to women's choice has been accompanied by a resurgence of interest in the late 1980s so that the percentage of home births in 1994 is now approaching 2% (Figure 1.3). This is encouraged by some women who feel that their ability to control events in childbirth is greater in the home than in the hospital. It has been reinforced by the Department of Health philosophy much of which is summed up in *Changing Childbirth*[11]. This document, issued in 1993, did not actually advocate home deliveries but certainly encouraged women to be offered a full choice which included home delivery with unbiased advice being given by the professionals. This utopian ideal of an unbiased professional is hard to find; some idea of these biases appears later in this report.

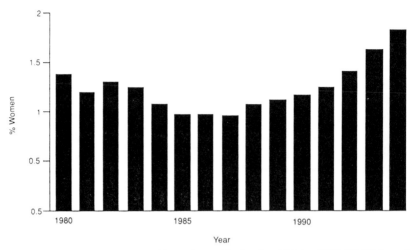

Figure 1.3 Percentage of maternities at home, England and Wales 1980–94 (Office of Populations, Censuses and Surveys)*

Several studies have been performed about women's attitudes and wishes for home birth. Usually the women examined are divided sharply into three groups: those who had no babies before, those who had babies in hospital and those who had delivered at home. Of the group with no previous experience, it would seem that between 5% and 15% of women would be interested in considering a home birth[12] if the facilities were available and adequate. Among those who had a baby before, those who had a home birth were very heavily in favour of a repeat performance while those who had a hospital delivery mostly wanted to go back there.

As well as the aspects of safety and woman's choice, financial constraints have been used as an argument against any domiciliary obstetric revival and any financial cuts must be overcome if it is to succeed. Without it we may have to revert to the past as predicted by Foster[13] from the Social Policy unit in Manchester:

> ...and since an underfunded NHS is equally unlikely to be able to provide the highest level of personal care and attention now demanded by more affluent consumers, we may well see, in the not too distant future, a return, albeit on a small scale, to a traditional class split within maternity care. Middle and upper class women may increasingly exercise the privilege of the true market place and opt out of NHS to alternate private maternity care services designed to give them the type of birth they desire in the place of their

choice. Meanwhile poor women will continue to go into the financially perilous NHS hospitals to give birth with less and less personal care and attention as the costs of the service, apart from the high technology systems insisted on by obstetricians, are pared to the bone. These women will probably continue to assume that discomforts they endure are a price well worth paying for the increased safety offered by modern obstetrical practices.

CONCLUSIONS

The history of home births is like so many other aspects of social history, a movement that has been driven by opinion rather than being evidence based. Birth at home was once the only choice; then alternatives emerged and many were secondarily sponsored by pressure groups of doctors and others. It has caused much debate, each side considering the other to be intransigent and protagonists proclaiming that they were advocating the best for women.

It is probably wise to let women be fully informed and educated about birth and its potential pleasures and problems; let them make their own risk assessments with guidance based on impartial information. When the woman's and her partner's decision has been made with proper consultation, the professionals should provide a service to cover what the women are seeking in their birth place rather than try to strait-jacket their ideas into rigid moulds laid down by one or other group of past protagonists.

REFERENCES

1. Chamberlain, G.V.P. (1996). Obstetrics in ancient Egypt. *St George's Hospital Medical School Gazette*, **103**, 6–8
2. Smelley, W. (1752). *Treatise on the Theory & Practice of Midwifery*, pp. 198–204. (London: D Wilson)
3. British College of Obstetricians and Gynaecologists (1936). *Memorandum on the Reorganisation of the Maternity Services*, p. 77. (London: BCOG)
4. British Medical Association (1936). The BMA and Maternity Services. *Br. Med. J.*, **1**, 656
5. National Birthday Trust Fund (1936). *Maternal Welfare – Analgesics for Moral Cases*. (London: NBTF)
6. Royal College of Obstetricians and Gynaecologists (1944). *A National Maternity Service*. (London: RCOG)
7. Cranbrook, Lord (1959). *Report on the Maternity Services*. (London: HMSO)

8. Peel, J. (1970). *Domiciliary Midwifery and Availability of Hospital Beds.* (London: HMSO)

9. Tew, M. (1977). Where to be born. *New Soc.*, **39**, 120–1

10. Royal College of Midwives (1987). *Towards a Healthy Nation.* (London: RCM)

11. Department of Health (1993). *Changing Childbirth.* (London: HMSO)

12. Campbell, R and Macfarlane, A. (1994). *Where to be Born?* (Oxford: National Perinatal Epidemiology Unit)

13. Foster, P. (1995). *Women and the Health Care Industry.* (Nottingham: Open University Press)

2

Organization of the study

At the beginning of 1993, the general committee of the National Birthday Trust Fund (NBTF) agreed to mount a study into home births. Professor Chamberlain was appointed the director and he set up a Steering group including representatives from both professional and consumer bodies. They had several meetings to consider the proposal and advise on specific issues. The Scientific Committee of the NBTF helped at this stage and later with the planning and progress of the study from its conception. Three directors were then appointed: Professor Geoffrey Chamberlain, Chairman of the NBTF Scientific Committee, Ann Wraight, a research midwife and Dr Patricia Crowley, a Dublin obstetrician with experience in epidemiology. Sarah Reed was appointed in August 1993 as secretary to the project and assistant to the Midwife Director. Dr Janet Peacock, a medical statistician at St George's Hospital Medical School, gave statistical advice. Professor Ann Oakley, a sociologist and member of the NBTF Scientific Committee, helped and analysed the follow-up survey, writing a chapter in the report. Jane Henderson and Dr Miranda Mugford analysed the economic implications of the information shown in the study and also provided a chapter for the report.

AIMS AND OBJECTIVE OF THE STUDY

The two primary aims of the NBTF study were originally:

(1)   To obtain a contemporary account of booked home births from midwives and from the women having babies in the UK during the year 1994.

(2)   To assess the outcome of those who planned to give birth at home compared to those who planned to give birth in hospital. This was to include physical measures, opinions and views of both the professionals and the women.

Objective

To perform a confidential prospective study of all women who were recruited at 37 weeks' gestation having been booked for home birth irrespective of where the birth took place. Those planning home births were matched with women of similar background and resident locality in age group, parity and obstetrical history, who at 37 weeks had planned to have their baby in hospital to provide a matched control group. Thus, entry to the study was well before the events of birth occurred and so it was hoped to remove the bias introduced by what happened in labour and delivery.

STUDY DESIGN

Liaison

Notification of the proposed study produced general agreement from the Health Departments of the four countries of the UK, England, Wales, Scotland and Northern Ireland. A short summary of the project was then sent to all Local Supervising Authorities along with a request for permission to contact all Supervisors of Midwives to gain their support and assistance. This was usually readily given. The Royal College of Midwives, the Royal College of Obstetricians and Gynaecologists and the Royal College of General Practitioners were also consulted. Much support and enthusiasm for this Enquiry into Home Births was expressed by all those contacted.

Supervisors of Midwives were chosen as contact persons in each District Health Authority for they liaise with all midwives employed in their area whether they work in the hospital, the community, or are independent. Thus they would be in a unique position to co-ordinate the data collection, for supervision of midwifery is statutory. All midwives must notify their intention to practise annually to the Local Supervising Authority through their Supervisors of Midwives. Of 282 Supervisors of Midwives, some with responsibility for the supervision of midwives within GP units as well as the parent hospital, 273 (97%) agreed to take part. Several of the nine Supervisors of Midwives who declined gave reasons which included that other local surveys or audits were already taking place in their areas of responsibility and they felt that one more set of data collection would put too much strain on the midwives' work-load or even cause a diminution of effort into the pre-existing studies.

From autumn 1993 to spring 1994, various Survey Directors attended 19 meetings to publicize the study, explain the practicalities and the reasons for some aspects, e.g. prospective registration to diminish bias. They met with groups of supervisors, midwives, GPs and obstetricians in England, Northern Ireland, Scotland and Wales. Articles were published in midwifery and medical journals and commentaries were written in the national press.

Method

All four countries of the UK were invited to take part in this study. The appropriate research instrument for this size of population was a postal questionnaire survey and success of the Survey would rest on an efficient postal service. The dedication of local midwives was essential while we also needed good communication and support of the NBTF Survey office.

The postal questionnaire Survey has advantages and disadvantages. Cost is lower compared with telephone or personal interviews due to a saving in time and travel. However, the respondents can experience a feeling of anonymity and there is less pressure for an immediate response to the question although it removes the risk of interviewer-bias influencing response. The reduced response rate is recognized as a major disadvantage; reports of response of about 50% are common if no reminder is sent to the respondents. The response rate is important since it is one of the indices of data quality control in a survey. There can be possible bias from non-responders for they may be at the extremes of the range from either end of the spectrum of opinion. By recruiting well before the event, at 37 weeks, we had hoped to reduce bias. We also strived for complete reporting among those recruited to the study and achieved an almost 98% response.

Once the questionnaires and notes of guidance had been tested locally with colleagues and volunteer postnatal mothers, two pilot studies were conducted, in the health districts of St George's Hospital in London and James Paget Hospital in Norfolk. The questionnaires were revised and despatched to the Supervisors of Midwives in the autumn of 1993. They were asked to discuss the study with local midwives and to seek their support and help. It was stressed that participation was entirely voluntary, so giving both the individual midwives and the women having babies the chance to refuse to take part at any time.

Throughout 1994, every midwife caring for a woman booked for home birth was issued with the relevant questionnaires by her Supervisor of Midwives and asked to discuss the study with each woman booked for a home birth by around 37 weeks' gestation, inviting her to take part. If the woman agreed, then the midwife was asked to identify another woman in her practice who matched the home birth mother but who had planned to have her baby in hospital. If the latter task proved to be impossible, the midwives were still encouraged to collect data from the planned home births; this was a notable problem for the majority of independent midwives who are involved in few hospital-booked births (221 in the home and only 18 in the hospital registered in this study). Notification of the women's names would then be made to the NBTF Survey office. This could be done by sending the relevant form or by telephoning the office with the information. A direct telephone line and an answerphone at the Survey office facilitated contact at any time in the 24 hours.

The decision not to place strict criteria on the selection of controls was made in the light of the results of the pilot studies. The availability of home birth varies greatly throughout the UK with the result that in some areas all women are given the choice of place of birth whereas in others only parous women with no previous or present problems are allowed to opt for home birth. It was therefore decided to ask the midwives to select as a control a woman who fulfilled criteria locally in a ranking order – the woman should live in the same locality as the home birth woman; be in the same age group (within 5 years); primigravida matched with primigravida and multigravida matched with multigravida; similar obstetric background in the case of multiparae. Those in the control group should have already planned and booked to have their babies in hospital.

REGISTRATION OF RESPONDENTS

The importance of registering the women well before labour started was stressed to the Supervisors of Midwives. The researchers were dependent on the midwives inviting all women planning home births to take part and also choosing other women planning hospital births as controls well before labour and to demonstrate that this had been done by registration at the Survey office. The results then would not show bias, for women were selected long before outcome was known. This extra task, an added burden on the midwives, was sometimes forgotten although letters to remind them of the aims of registration were sent twice. Despite this, 415 questionnaires had to be discarded because names had not been registered prospectively.

When the study closed, it was noted that no questionnaire (from either midwife or woman) had been received for over 900 women who had been registered as willing to take part in the Survey. In an effort to exclude non-participation due to poor outcome rather than other reasons, the Supervisors of Midwives were again contacted and asked to provide some basic data on these women so that these could be examined for bias. Neither the women nor the individual midwives were contacted since they had been assured that participation was voluntary. They could change their minds about their wish to participate at any time and some did.

Of the 948 women registered in the Survey but with no questionnaires from themselves or their midwives, 785 forms of the briefer information set were received from Supervisors – an 83% response rate. Thus the majority of the Supervisors of Midwives were able to provide some statistical information, although they could not give attitudinal data. Four Supervisors of Midwives replied that they were unable to provide any details on any of the women who had not responded.

Comparisons of the distributions on some key variables were made between the population in the main sample, the extra data from the non-responders and the national figures published by the Office for National Statistics. The results are discussed in Chapter 3.

ETHICS APPROVAL

Since the early NBTF surveys, ethics committees had become established and had to be consulted about data collection in their locality. Since no National or Regional Ethics Committees (apart from Northern Ireland) existed, the Supervisor of Midwives in every district had to seek approval, on behalf of the research team, for the data collection to take place locally. This was requested in the Autumn of 1993.

The process varied greatly throughout the four countries. In some districts, the Chairman of the Ethics Committee, having read the proposal, gave approval without further discussion; in others, the Supervisor of Midwives was asked to complete a form which would be presented at the next meeting. Eleven Supervisors of Midwives did not feel they had sufficient information in order to complete these forms and so posted them on for the attention of the co-ordinator at the NBTF office who put in a direct request. Eighteen Committees requested copies of each questionnaire, notes of guidance, summary sheets and protocols and asked for enough for each Committee member. A further 15 Committee Chairmen requested answers to specific questions raised at a meeting when the study protocol was discussed. Since it was impossible for a member of the research team to attend each meeting personally, any questions had to be answered in writing resulting in further delay in the approval process.

There was no uniformity in the Committees' examinations of the study nor indeed in their concerns. These included issues relating to Data Protection, confidentiality, ability of respondents to opt out at any time, access to statisticians, as well as specific questions such as ethnicity. Each of these was identified by only one Committee. One gave approval to the study in principle but requested that the colour of the questionnaires be changed. They did not like the idea that the women's questionnaires were pink (home) and blue (hospital). They felt that this might lead to confusion for women in the home group who gave birth to boys and for women in the hospital group who gave birth to girls. Happily, all the Local Research Ethics Committees eventually gave the study their approval, although 15 had not considered it by the start date of the Survey resulting in no data being collected in these districts for the first few weeks of the year.

DATA COLLECTION

The data collection began on 1 January 1994 and continued until 31 December 1994. Following the births of the babies in home and hospital, both women and midwives were asked to complete questionnaires and return them to the Survey office. In some areas, a Supervisor of Midwives took responsibility for the co-ordination of the total data collection, receiving completed questionnaires and following up non-responders before returning the forms to the Survey office. In most locations, however, each midwife took responsibility for her own forms, sending them directly to the office. Each mother had a Business Reply envelope enclosed in her questionnaire so that she had the option of posting it back without involving either the midwife or the Supervisor. Table 2.1 shows the flow of the questionnaires between the respondents and the NBTF Survey office.

Questions asked in the midwife's form related to background information on the women themselves, their past obstetrical history and outcome of this pregnancy; also some information was asked on the

Table 2.1 Despatch and return of questionnaires (NBTF Home Births Survey 1994)

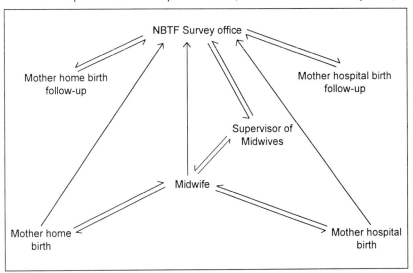

equipment available for the home births. The mothers were requested to describe their experiences and satisfaction with their care. A separate questionnaire was prepared for women who had a stillbirth or whose baby died soon after birth. Previous NBTF surveys had highlighted the fact that women who lost a baby do not want to be excluded from giving their views[1].

A random sample (20%) of the women in both home and hospital-booked groups were sent a follow-up questionnaire when their baby was 6–8 weeks old to detect any shift in attitude with the passage of time. These forms were posted directly to the woman's home. The sampling was done by the computer program Clinstat which was written by Professor Martin Bland, Professor of Medical Statistics at St George's Hospital Medical School.

UNPLANNED HOME BIRTHS

The NBTF Survey had been planned to examine booked home deliveries only but the Directors were persuaded by various interested groups that this was an opportunity to assess something of unplanned home births. Obviously the same prospective careful plans were inappropriate and so a separate short anonymous questionnaire on unplanned home births was prepared and sent out to be completed by the Supervisors of Midwives.

The women and individual midwives were not involved in this section for it was not really part of the planned study. Application for Ethics Committee approval was also made for this.

All questionnaires are reproduced in the Appendix.

PROCESS OF THE DATA ANALYSIS

On arrival at the Survey office, each questionnaire was checked against the registration lists and then rendered anonymous by the removal of all personal and geographical details. A unique survey number was issued to each form, the open questions were coded and the data were entered on to computer.

The Scottish data collection was co-ordinated in Edinburgh by Dr Tricia Murphy-Black and Katherine Pinkerton; the NBTF is grateful for the assistance they gave. The Scottish Home and Health Department had also been considering conducting a similar study on home and DOMINO births in Scotland. They agreed to link with the NBTF study, agreeing to amend their data collection forms to include certain questions that the NBTF asked. Thus the information from Scotland was rendered uniform with the NBTF study. When the Survey closed, the Scottish data were sent to the NBTF Survey office so that they could be merged with the main data sets.

The SPSS system was used to access and analyse the data. Examination of individual files was done on a personal computer in the Survey office, but the merging of the files (women's questionnaires + midwives' questionnaires + follow-up questionnaires) and further analyses of these very large data sets were done on the Sun computer at St George's Hospital Medical School. The NBTF is grateful for the help given by Richard Hulkhory in the computer unit there.

Since this was purely a descriptive study, analysis of the data was by simple frequency distributions and cross-tabulations. Subsets of the population were examined, e.g. women who intended to give birth at home and achieved that, were separated from those who planned to be at home but had to be transferred to hospital for the birth. Statistical procedures, therefore, were used only if the clinical significance of the results was in doubt. χ^2 tests were used to investigate the association between categorical variables such as place of birth and social class. Dr Janet Peacock advised the research team on the need and benefits of such further statistical analysis.

Table 2.2 Returned questionnaires (NBTF Home Births Survey 1994)

Questionnaire	*Number*	
Planned home births		
Questionnaires from both women and midwives	4116	
Questionnaires from women only	887	
Questionnaires from midwives only	589	
Minimal data from Supervisors of Midwives	379	
Total women on whom we had information	5971	
Total women registered to join the study	6044	(98.7% response rate)
Planned hospital births		
Questionnaires from both women and midwives	2733	
Questionnaires from women only	773	
Questionnaires from midwives only	619	
Minimal data from Supervisors of Midwives	406	
Total women on whom we had information	4634	
Total women registered to join the study	4724	(98% response rate)
Follow-up (home)	855	
Follow-up (hospital)	645	
Discarded (data received but women not registered prospectively)	415	
Discarded (late arrivals)	12	
Unplanned home births	1600	

PARTICIPATION OF RESPONDENTS

The final data for the main study were collected up to the last day of 1994 and for the follow-up study up to the last day of February 1995. The entering of the data closed finally in May 1995 for by then the flood had become a trickle. Twelve questionnaires only were returned after the closure date. One mother completed and returned her questionnaire on 15 July 1996 when her baby was 2 years old. Table 2.2 lists the number of completed questionnaires received and entered, along with those not used for various reasons.

CONCLUSIONS

The co-operation of Health Departments and management structure is helpful if sought; the professionals were very helpful at all grades but there are signs of questionnaire fatigue. We are all auditing and assaying aspects of the Health Services in the UK in a time of great self-examination. Hence, another detailed questionnaire survey is greeted with modified pleasure. The diversity of local ethics committees is a problem for national surveys but given a long enough lead-up time they can all be consulted. The NBTF is again, for the sixth time, grateful to the midwives for their help in collecting data.

There were 12 352 babies born at home (planned and unplanned) in the UK in 1994. The number of completed questionnaires received in this Survey which related to home births, from mother or midwife or both, was 5592. Details on a further 379 forms completed by the Supervisors on women, registered in the study and planning to give birth at home but who had not returned their questionnaires, brings the total to 5971.

Data on 7571 women who gave birth at home (5971 planned and 1600 unplanned) were collected in this Survey – 61.3% of all home births in the UK in 1994. Although this is a large sample, it still indicates the decline in acceptance rates for NBTF studies since 1970. There appear to be three reasons for this:

(1) The increasing call on both professionals and consumers to fill forms to meet the needs of the health services and maternity care providers in particular, as the service is being increasingly audited and researched.

(2) The late start of the data collection in some districts since Local Research Ethics Committee approval had not been received.

(3) No reminder letters were sent to any of the respondents at any stage of this Survey, for all participating women having babies and mid-wives were volunteers and the NBTF did not wish to appear to coerce voluntary action. This practice had been followed in previous NBTF studies. The response rates of the six NBTF surveys since 1946 can be seen in Table 2.3.

Table 2.3 Response rates of NBTF Surveys, 1946–94

Year	Study	Respondents	Reminder letters/ telephone calls	Response rate (%)
1946	Maternity in Great Britain	supervisors of midwives	yes	90 (approx.)
1958	Perinatal Mortality	midwives	yes	92 (approx.)
1970	British Births Vol. I & II	midwives	yes	98 (approx.)
1984	Place of Birth	supervisors of midwives	yes	99.1
1990	Pain Relief in Labour	mothers partners midwives GPs obstetricians anaesthetists paediatricians	no	66
	Follow-up	mothers	yes	82
1994	Home births Recruitment	mothers	no	61 (approx.)
	Response of recruited	midwives and mothers		98 (approx.)
	Follow-up	mothers	no	83

Thirty-eight per cent of the women in both groups wrote comments on their questionnaires in the main study. In the follow-up study almost three-quarters of the home birth group (73%) and almost half (49%) of the hospital group gave comments. In this section, the partners were also invited to give comments. Twenty-eight per cent of the partners in the home birth group and 5% of the hospital group took up this invitation. Both groups of midwives were asked to write comments. Only 6% of the home birth sample and 4% of the hospital sample did so. The majority of the comments were constructive and positive and some have been used to illustrate the report.

REPORT OF THE FINDINGS

To maintain confidentiality, no data analysis has been made at District Health Authority (DHA) level. DHA data could easily be describing information about all births in the district and if these were few it could breach confidentiality. Data from each unit have been grouped into regional and national data.

Some of the findings of the individual units were analysed separately and sent to the relevant key Supervisor of Midwives for her interest and use. Issues included women's satisfaction with care, options offered to her on place of birth, or transfer to hospital. National figures were tabulated so that local results could be compared with these.

The first presentation of the findings was made to the Royal College of Midwives on October 3 1996 and to the Royal College of Obstetricians and Gynaecologists on November 8 1996. Many other meetings of midwives, obstetricians and consumers were addressed after this.

The report itself was mostly drafted by the three directors. Like many NBTF reports it aims to give the data with background to place them in context. We have tried not to let our professional opinions enter but a report of numbers only would be dry and tax the reader. Hence we have used some opinions of the women, their partners and the midwives for they were there. Other observations come from secondary sources chosen by the authors.

Table 2.4 Timetable of the NBTF Home Births Study (NBTF Home Births Survey 1994)

	1993 JJASOND	1994 JFMAMJJASOND	1995 JFMAMJJASOND	1996 JFMAMJJ
Communication with all involved	————————	————————	————————	————————
Advertisement of study	—			
Preparation of questionnaires	—			
Pilot studies (2)	—			
Despatch of questionnaires				
main sample		————		
follow-up sample		————		
Registration of respondents		————		
Coding of questionnaires		————		
Data entering		————		
Data analysis and editing			———	
Writing report				———
Feedback of local results to individual Supervisors of Midwives				—

SUMMARY

This study was a descriptive, prospective survey involving women who had planned to give birth at home and a control group of women, matched in age, parity and residence, who had planned to have their babies in hospital. Information was also received from midwives who were present at the births. Some additional information about unplanned home birth was also solicited.

Although the preliminary preparations for the study started at the beginning of 1993, the main process began in June of that year with the appointment of the Midwife Director. Table 2.4 demonstrates the stages of the study with overlap in some cases. The total funding for the 3-year project was provided by the NBTF.

The response rate of those who did register was high (98.7%). The findings of this large sample of women giving birth in the UK in 1994 are illuminating. Their comments are constructive and many have been included in the following chapters to highlight some of the findings. The study describes the experiences, the satisfaction and the outcomes of the respondents relating to their babies' births at home, comparing them with institutions throughout the UK in 1994.

Several women commented on the need for such a study and expressed a hope that the findings would provide useful information on the place of birth. The following is an example from a mother who gave birth at home:

> I found completing a survey like this very useful as a way of thinking about my labour and going over it afterwards – a very necessary part of coming to terms with the intensity, the trauma, the excitement of the experience.

REFERENCE

1. Chamberlain, G., Wraight, A. and Steer, P. (1993). *Pain and its Relief in Childbirth*. (London: Churchill Livingstone)

3

Profile of women and the survey

Many obstetricians have an ambition to carry out a randomized controlled trial of home versus hospital birth, where women are randomly allocated to the intended place of birth. Bias and confounding variables would be eliminated by the process of randomization so that any differences in outcome are more likely to be attributable to the effects of place of birth. Such a trial is, and may remain, a dream.

Dowswell and co-workers[1] argue that, while the numbers required to perform a trial of sufficient power to answer questions about safety of home birth are prohibitive, a smaller trial, measuring outcomes other than safety, would be feasible. Views about the safety of home versus hospital birth are so firmly held by both child-bearing women and by health care professionals that few are likely to achieve the state of neutrality necessary to participate comfortably in a trial[2]. In their pilot study in Leeds, Dowswell and co-workers[1] found that 71 women out of a population of about 500 were eligible for randomization. Of these, only 11 agreed to take part.

The present study had, by necessity, to rely on a more pragmatic but scientifically less robust design. Women planning to give birth at home were prospectively asked to join the study. Thus a pair of selection biases could have been introduced – first, that of those midwives who were willing to ask women to participate and to perform the data collection and secondly the women who having already decided on a home birth, were prepared to join in and allow those labours to be documented. To this group were matched for age and parity, as described in Chapter 2, women planning a hospital birth selected by the investigating midwife from her

Table 3.1 Analysis of participants by age

| | NBTF Study 1994 | | | | England and Wales 1994 | | | |
| | Planned home (n = 5003) | | Planned hospital (n = 3506) | | Home* (n = 11 852) | | Hospital (n = 647 692) | |
Age	n	%	n	%	n	%	n	%
<20 years	12	0.2	30	0.9	220	1.8	41 820	6.5
20–29 years	1841	37.6	1403	41.0	5208	44.0	361 992	55.9
30–39 years	2900	59.3	1931	56.5	6182	52.2	233 438	36.0
40–49 years	138	2.8	56	1.6	242	2.0	10 442	1.6
Not known/ recorded	112		86		0		0	

*The national data are of births at home (planned and unplanned) while the Survey data are of planned only

Table 3.2 Analysis of participants by parity

| | NBTF Study 1994 | | | | England and Wales 1994 | | | |
| | Planned home (n = 5003) | | Planned hospital (n = 3506) | | Home* (n = 8447) | | Hospital (n = 436 589) | |
Parity	n	%	n	%	n	%	n	%
0	791	15.9	553	15.8	869	10.3	173 319	39.7
1,2,3	3996	80.2	2875	82.2	7170	84.9	250 263	57.3
≥4	199	3.9	71	2.0	408	4.8	13 007	3.0
Not known/ recorded	17		7		0		0	

*National figures relate only to babies born within marriage and to both planned and unplanned home births

practice – obviously a geographically similar group. A comparison of the characteristics of the two groups of women in the study allows us to assess the success of the matching process and to relate the characteristics of these two subgroups of women to the overall obstetric population.

AGE, PARITY AND ETHNIC GROUP

In this National Birthday Trust Fund (NBTF) 1994 study, matching with respect to age and parity are shown in Tables 3.1 and 3.2. Both groups of women participating in the study were older and the hospital group was of higher parity than the general population of women in the UK in 1994. Study participants from the four London regions were older than those in the rest of the country. Sixty-nine per cent of London women choosing home birth were 30 years of age or older.

Table 3.3 Analysis of participants by ethnic origin reported by women (NBTF Home Births Survey 1994)

| | *Home (n = 5003)* | | *Hospital (n = 3506)* | |
	n	%	n	%
White	4886	97.7	3447	98.3
West Indian	33	0.7	23	0.7
Indian	13	0.3	10	0.3
Pakistani	3	<0.1	7	0.2
Bangladeshi	0	—	2	0.1
African	13	0.3	3	0.1
Other	34	0.7	6	0.2
Not answered	21	0.4	8	0.2

Table 3.4 Woman's occupation reported by women (NBTF Home Births Survey 1994)

| | *Home (n = 5003)* | | Hospital (*n* = 3506) | |
Social class	n	%	n	%
I & II	1966	39.2	859	24.5
III	1771	35.4	1733	49.4
IV, V & Armed Forces	228	4.6	282	8.1
Housewife	1038	20.8	632	18.0

There was no great ethnic origin difference between the two groups in the Survey but ethnic minorities were small in the whole study (2% among both home and hospital-planned births). There were few who booked for home birth and so the control group followed this trend (see Table 3.3).

SOCIAL CLASS AND EDUCATION

Women giving birth at home were of higher social class using either their own or their partner's occupation as an index (Tables 3.4 and 3.5; Figure 3.1). They had completed more years of full-time education compared with those delivering in hospital (Table 3.6 and Figure 3.2). There was no difference in the proportion of women working outside the home, but of the 80% of women who were employed, a significantly higher proportion of the home birth group were in professional or skilled occupations.

In addition to these important differences in social class and educational attainment, women intending to give birth at home were

31

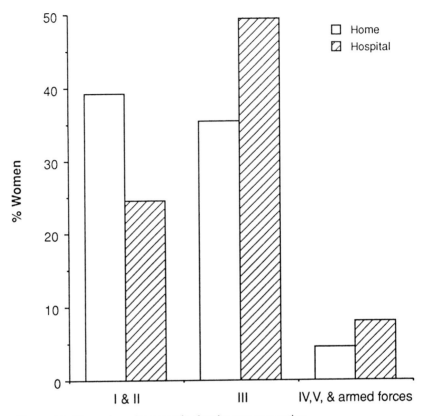

Figure 3.1 Women's socioeconomic class by own occupation

Table 3.5 Partner's occupation reported by women (NBTF Home Births Survey 1994)

Social class	Home (n = 5003)		Hospital (n = 3506)		England & Wales (n = 582 600)	
	n	%	n	%	n	%
I & II	2122	42.7	1122	32.2	195 600	33.6
III	2023	40.7	1709	49.0	263 400	45.2
IV, V & Armed Forces	495	10.0	501	14.3	123 600	21.2
Unemployed/student	334	6.6	157	4.5	—	
Not known/recorded	29		17		—	

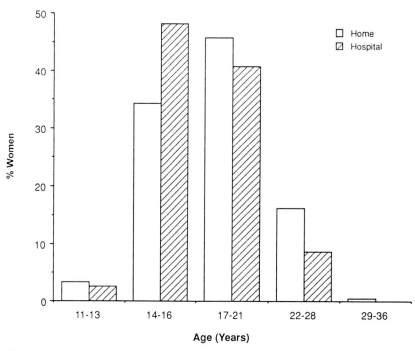

Figure 3.2 Age of completion of education

Table 3.6 Age of completion of education reported by women (NBTF Home Births Survey 1994)

Age (years)	Home (n = 5003)		Hospital (n = 3506)	
	n	%	n	%
11–13	163	3.3	91	2.6
14–16	1709	34.3	1684	48.2
17–21	2281	45.8	1421	40.7
22–28	805	16.2	299	8.6
29–36	26	0.5	—	
Not known/recorded	19		11	

significantly different with respect to their intended method of infant feeding. Seventy-nine per cent of women who intended to give birth at home planned to breast-feed compared with 57% of those who planned a hospital birth (3949/5003 home compared with 2002/3506 hospital). This is consistent with the tendency for women of higher social class with more years of completed education to breast-feed[3]. This tendency may also be an indicator of more subtle differences in attitudes towards child-bearing and child rearing between the two groups such as self-confidence, and a

33

desire for autonomy and control. Chapters 5, 6 and 9 provide additional insights into some of these issues.

PAST OBSTETRIC HISTORY

In the study of planned home births 16% were nulliparae and 84% multiparae. Predictably, many of the women planning a home birth had experienced home birth before. Among parous women 31% had experienced at least one previous home birth compared with only 1% of those intending hospital birth.

There was no difference between the two groups of women with respect to perinatal mortality among previous children. The total perinatal mortality rate in all previous pregnancies was 4.6 per 1000 in the control group intending to deliver in hospital and 4.9 per 1000 in those intending to deliver at home. Those planning a home birth were an extremely low risk group. Only 1% had had a Caesarean section in the past compared with 3% of those planning a hospital birth. The low incidence of low birthweight among the previous babies of the home birth group – 2% compared with 3% of the hospital group and a national rate of 7% – is again indicative of an extremely low level of obstetric risk.

INDEX PREGNANCY

In addition to having a lower level of obstetric risk from the past obstetric history, women planning a home birth had fewer antepartum complications in the index pregnancy.

The differing incidence of hypertensive disorders of pregnancy may reflect a baseline difference between the two groups of women or an ascertainment bias associated with a greater number of hospital-based antenatal visits in this group intending hospital birth. However, since the recruitment time was by 37 weeks, some who originally had planned a home birth may have had a complication in earlier pregnancy so the booking plans changed and they never entered the Survey. Given the effect of psychosocial factors on blood pressure[4] it is possible that the increased amount of midwifery-led antenatal care experienced by the home birth group or the psychological benefits of anticipated home birth had a protective effect on the likelihood of showing pregnancy-induced hypertension. During a recent randomized trial of routine antenatal care by general practitioners and midwives compared with shared care led by obstetricians, the incidence of pregnancy-induced hypertension,

Table 3.7 Complications in current pregnancy reported by women (NBTF Home Births Survey 1994)

Problem	*Home (n = 5003)*		*Hospital (n = 3506)*	
	n	%	n	%
Hypertension	220	4.4	315	9.1
Pre-eclampsia	25	0.5	52	1.5
Diabetes	17	0.3	26	0.7
Vaginal bleeding	432	8.6	374	10.7
Not known/recorded	3		11	

pre-eclampsia and proteinuria was reduced in those allocated to antenatal care by general practitioners and midwives[5].

The two groups matched well for birthweight in the index pregnancy. The incidence of low birthweight, below 2500 g, was 1% in the group who planned home birth and 1% in the group who planned hospital birth, while 16% of those planning home birth gave birth to babies weighing over 4000 g compared with 16% of those planning hospital birth. However, among primigravidae, 14% of those intending home birth had babies greater than 4000 g compared with 10% of those planning hospital birth. This may reflect baseline characteristics of the two groups, variations in the incidence of hypertensive disorders with a variation in the rate of induction of labour.

COMPLETENESS OF THE SURVEY

This Survey depended upon the willingness of the midwives to invite women to join and the preparedness of the women themselves to take part in the Survey. We have expressed our thoughts about the returns (Chapter 2) and the degree to which the Survey population was representative. The analysis that we performed is on those women who, with their midwives, took part in a voluntary study. We are aware that amongst those who did not contribute there may be certain swings of behaviour or outcome.

The Survey basically compared those women who by 37 weeks had intended to have a home delivery with those who by the same gestation intended to give birth in hospital. As well as the analysis of groups defined by intent, we also analysed by actuality. For example, the women who having intended a home birth but ended with a Caesarean section obviously did not deliver at home but after transfer to hospital. Other events may be less obvious and so analysis by both intent and by actuality is assessed to reverse bias in the first and relate what happened to facilities in the second.

Table 3.8 The number of women registered prospectively in the study and the number of questionnaires returned (NBTF Home Births Survey 1994)

| | Intended place of birth | | | |
| | Home | | Hospital | |
	n	*%*	*n*	*%*
Enrolled in study	6044		4724	
Questionnaire from woman (total)	5003	82.8	3506	74.0
Questionnaire from midwife (total)	4705	77.8	3352	71.0
Questionnaire from either or both	5592	92.5	4228	89.5
Minimal data from Supervisors of Midwives	379	6.3	406	8.6
No data	73	1.2	90	1.9

Table 3.9 Returned questionnaires in each category of those who had planned their delivery site (NBTF Home Births Survey 1994)

	Planned and delivered at home	*Planned and delivered in hospital*	*Planned home but delivered in hospital*	*Planned hospital but delivered at home*
Midwife questionnaires	3922	3319	769	33
Mothers questionnaires	4191	3470	806	36

Table 3.8 shows the breakdown of all those who were registered in the NBTF Survey. Only 1% of the planned home group and 2% of the planned hospital group are unaccounted for. These women formed two major and four subgroups (Table 3.9). The first is those who intended to deliver at home and made firm plans for this by 37 weeks; they may be subdivided into those who gave birth at home and those who had to be transferred to hospital for delivery. The other major grouping, the controls, were those women who intended to deliver in hospital and had so booked by 37 weeks; the vast majority of these women achieved this but a small number did not get to the hospital in time for delivery – these made up the third and fourth subgroups planned hospital/delivered hospital and planned hospital/delivered elsewhere. There were questionnaires from midwives and the women themselves relating to each delivery and so the data on which this section is prepared come from denominators that vary slightly according to source examined.

Thus, of the 5003 women who planned a home birth, 806 did not achieve it (16%). Of the 3506 women who were the hospital-booked controls, only 33 did not deliver in hospital (1%). The number of questionnaires received from the mothers did not always match the number from the midwives but was close. This was a survey of the voluntary returns of women and midwives about planned deliveries and so these are considered in the following chapter. Any data collected on the unplanned home births are considered separately in Chapter 8.

WOMEN WHO WERE REGISTERED BUT WERE UNASSESSED

After delivery, a completed questionnaire was obtained from either a midwife or the woman herself or both in 92% of women intending home birth and in 89% of women intending hospital birth. A further questionnaire was sent to the Supervisor of Midwives to ascertain the fate of the 948 non-responders. The Supervisors were able to supply minimal data on the outcome of 785 (83%) comprising 379 women who intended home delivery and 406 who intended hospital birth leaving only 73 women from the home group and 90 from the hospital group for whom we have no data (Table 3.8), a completeness rate for those 6044 enrolling who planned home birth of 98.7%.

The validity of the study results is potentially threatened, both by selection bias and by exclusion bias. We have shown how the two groups registered in the study were matched for age and parity, but how the groups differed with respect to social class and education. Both *hard* outcomes such as mode of delivery and *soft* outcomes such as maternal satisfaction could be influenced either by these baseline differences or by the place of birth. Bias could also be introduced by exclusion from the final analysis of some of the women who registered for the study. Tables 3.10 and 3.11 and Figures 3.3 and 3.4 summarize the completeness of data collection.

Starting from the total number of women registered in the study there is a hierarchy of completeness from those whose outcome is completely documented by both a midwife's and a woman's questionnaire, to those for whom the Supervisor of Midwives supplied minimal data only. Only 1% of the home birth group and 2% of the hospital group are unaccounted for without even minimum outcome data. Many of these women may have been lost to follow-up for completely neutral reasons, such as moving house or inertia. However, we could not disregard the possibility that some women or midwives may have failed to complete questionnaires because of unsatisfactory outcomes.

A number of calculations were performed to assess the extent of any assessment bias. Among those who intended home birth, a number of major outcomes was reported in both woman's and midwife's

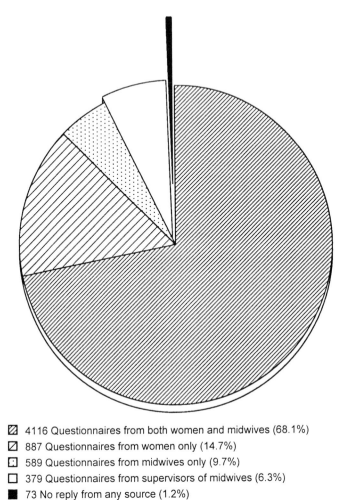

☒ 4116 Questionnaires from both women and midwives (68.1%)
☒ 887 Questionnaires from women only (14.7%)
⊡ 589 Questionnaires from midwives only (9.7%)
☐ 379 Questionnaires from supervisors of midwives (6.3%)
■ 73 No reply from any source (1.2%)

Figure 3.3 Returns of questionnaires – planned home births

questionnaires. The incidence of these outcomes is presented in Table 3.10.

This exercise indicates a reassuring consistency between outcomes based on the two questionnaires from the group who intended home birth. All five perinatal deaths reported by women were also reported by midwives. The consistency between the midwives' and women's questionnaires suggests that little bias is introduced by quoting outcomes derived from either of these subsets. Using the incidence rates derived

Table 3.10 Comparison of outcomes derived from various samples of women planning home birth (NBTF Home Births Survey 1994)

Outcome	Midwives		Women		Either	Minimal data		Any data	All enrolled	
	n	%	n	%		n	%		n	%
Hospital birth	769	16.3*	806	16.1	900–911*	166	43.8	1066–1077*	1066–1150	17.6–19.0**
Induction	216	4.6	206	4.1	229–257*	31	8.1*	260–288*	260–361	4.3–6.0**
Assisted delivery	115	2.4	121	2.4	134*	12	3.2*	146*	146–219	2.4–3.6**
Caesarean section	94	2.0	100	2.0	112*	24	6.3*	136*	136–209	2.3–3.5**
Perinatal death	5*		5*		5*	3*		8*	8–81 (1.3–13.4 per 1000)**	
Total	4705		5003		5592	379		5971	6044	

*Actual; **Estimated

Table 3.11 Comparison of outcomes derived from various samples of women planning hospital birth (NBTF Home Births Survey 1994)

Outcome	Midwives		Women		Either	Minimal data		Any data		All enrolled	
	n	%	n	%		n	%	n	%	n	%
Induction	613	18.3*	N/K		769**	13	3.1*	782	16.9**	782–872	16.4–18.5**
Assisted delivery	180	5.4*	N/K		228**	19	4.6*	247	5.3**	247–364	5.2–7.1**
Caesarean section	139	4.1*	N/K		173**	34	8.3*	207	4.5**	207–297	4.4–6.3**
Perinatal death	5*		5*		5*	1*		6*		6–128 (1.2–26 per 1000)**	
Total	3352		3506		4228	406		4634		4724	

*Actual; **Estimated; NK, not known

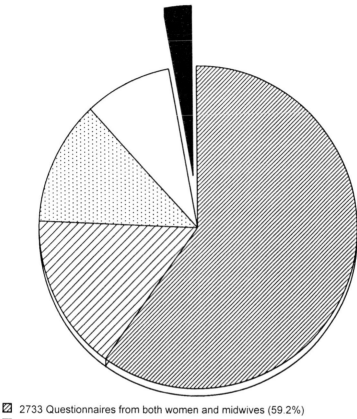

☑ 2733 Questionnaires from both women and midwives (59.2%)
☑ 773 Questionnaires from women only (16.7%)
☒ 619 Questionnaires from midwives only (13.4%)
☐ 406 Questionnaires from supervisors of midwives (8.8%)
■ 90 No reply from any source (1.9%)

Figure 3.4 Returns of questionnaires – planned hospital births

from the woman's and midwife's questionnaires, the incidence of these outcomes was derived for the 5592 women on whom either or both questionnaires is available. The minimal data supplied by the midwifery supervisors were added to this to calculate the outcome for all 5971 women on whom any data are available. The addition of the minimal data supplied for non-responders has little effect on any outcome with the exception of perinatal death. The final column in Table 3.10 estimates the minimum and maximum rates for the various outcomes assuming either none or all of the 73 women on whom we have no data had this outcome. It is clear that the size of the potential bias arising from incomplete data collection is small when frequently occurring outcomes, such as transfer to hospital, induction of labour, Caesarean section, are concerned. Rare outcomes such as perinatal death are invalidated.

Unfortunately, the exercise cannot be repeated for women who planned hospital birth as women were not asked about method of delivery in a planned site (Table 3.11), only the midwives. The rate for these outcomes calculated for those who supplied any data is an estimate based on the rate from the midwives' questionnaire. The only outcome requested from both women and midwives in this arm is perinatal death. As with those planning home birth, a midwife's questionnaire and a woman's questionnaire were received for all five perinatal deaths in the group intending hospital birth. As there were 90 women in the hospital-booked group on whom no data whatsoever are available, the estimated maximum possible rate for all the outcomes is higher.

The data presented in Tables 3.10 and 3.11 indicate that incomplete data collection is not a major source of bias where the main outcomes are concerned. This is particularly the case with respect to those planning home birth where data collection is more complete.

We had recognized from the outset that this study did not have the power to detect any differences in perinatal death between women intending home or hospital birth. Tables 3.10 and 3.11 show how these rare outcomes are completely invalidated by even small deficits in data collection. It is therefore essential that no conclusions are drawn from the figures relating to perinatal death.

CONCLUSIONS

At entry into the study, women booking a home delivery and therefore their controls were privileged socially and biologically. Compared with the overall population, they had both experienced a low rate of adverse obstetric outcome in the past and had relatively few adverse events in the current pregnancy. In all respects, those planning to deliver at home were an even lower risk group than the controls for they were more affluent women with a superior educational background, and a higher rate of intended breast-feeding. Their lower incidence of previous Caesarean section and hypertensive disorders in the current pregnancy predisposed them to a lower rate of intervention and adverse outcome irrespective of the place of birth. This analysis is capable of identifying only the more easily measurable obstetric and demographic characteristics of the study population. In a society where less than 2% of women plan to give birth at home, it is inevitable that those who do so differ from their child-bearing peers in other more subtle but fundamental ways.

It would seem that the group of women who registered but did not respond by returning a questionnaire had a worse experience with an increase in interventions and more adverse outcomes. They are small in numbers and Tables 3.10 and 3.11 show that their addition would not have made a big difference to most of the proportions shown in our Survey. Their comments would probably have been useful and could have added to our knowledge of what women feel about home births particularly when unexpected problems arise.

This was a volunteer study of women who had already booked their place of delivery and were recruited well before the childbirth. Acceptance rates (61%) were not high but response rates of those who volunteered were very gratifying (98%). The women who elected for home births were from a high socioeconomic echelon and were educationally and biologically different from the controls planning a hospital birth.

REFERENCES

1. Dowswell, T., Thornton, J.G., Hewison, J. and Lilford, R.J.L. (1996). Should there be a trial of home versus hospital delivery in the United Kingdom? Measuring outcomes other than safety is feasible. *Br. Med. J.*, **321**,753–7

2. Lilford, R. and Jackson, I. (1995). Equipoise and the ethics of randomisation. *J. Roy. Soc. Med.*, **88**, 552–9

3. Martin, J. (1988). *Infant Feeding 1985*. (London: HM Stationery Office)

4. Little, B.C., Hayworth, J., Benson, P., Hall, F., Beard, R.W. and Dewhurst, J. (1984). Treatment of hypertension in pregnancy by relaxation and biofeedback. *Lancet*, **1**, 865–7

5. Tucker, J.S., Hall, M.H., Howie, P., Reid, M.E., Barbour, R.S., Florey, C. du V. and McIlwaine, G. (1996). Should obstetricians see women with normal pregnancies? A multicentre randomised controlled trial of routine antenatal care by general practitioners and midwives compared with shared care led by obstetricians. *Br. Med. J.*, **316**, 554–9

4

The birth

In this section of the report, the 3922 women who had planned and delivered at home are compared with 3319 who had booked for hospital delivery and did deliver there. Additional comparisons are made also with the 769 women who had planned to deliver at home by 37 weeks but actually delivered in hospital. The group of hospital booked/home delivered contained only 33 women and was too small for detailed analysis.

The range of planned home deliveries is shown in Table 4.1 and Figure 4.1. South Western and South East Thames share 22% of all the planned home deliveries reported while East Anglia, Oxford and Wessex returns were 6–8%. Generally the more northern regions are low – Mersey 2%, Yorkshire 4% and Northern 2%. The Celtic crescent reported Wales as 6%, Scotland 4% and Northern Ireland 1%, the lowest proportion of any region.

INDUCTION OF LABOUR AND RUPTURE OF MEMBRANES

An answer to the question to the midwives about whether labour was induced showed that while only 0.2% of women in the home planned/home delivered group were induced, this occurred in 19% of the hospital planned/hospital delivered women, a hundredfold difference. Among the home planned/hospital delivered group induction rates were even higher, at 29%.

In answer to the questions about augmentation of labour with rupture of the membranes by the midwife or doctor once labour had started, the

Table 4.1 The regional distribution of home planned/home delivered births reported by midwives (NBTF Home Births Survey 1994)

Region	n	% Study total
Northern	88	2.2
Yorkshire	162	4.1
Trent	202	5.2
East Anglia	316	8.0
North West Thames	304	7.7
North East Thames	229	5.8
South East Thames	414	10.5
South West Thames	235	5.9
Wessex	241	6.1
Oxford	251	6.4
South Western	445	11.3
West Midlands	295	7.5
Mersey	96	2.5
North Western	217	5.5
Northern Ireland	23	0.6
Scotland	158	4.0
Wales	246	6.2
Total	3922	

procedure was performed in 1276 (33%) home planned/home delivered women. Only 7% had this done at 4 cm cervical dilatation or less; 46% had the rupture performed between 5 and 8 cm and in the remainder (47%), the cervices were 9 cm or at full dilatation (Figure 4.2). Thus membrane rupture was later in this group than in the other groups. In the hospital planned/hospital delivered group 52% had their membranes ruptured in labour. Figure 4.3 shows a quarter had their membranes ruptured at or before 4 cm dilatation and another third before 9 cm. Similar proportions occurred in the home planned/hospital delivered group with 51% of women reporting having membranes ruptured artificially during labour and the distribution of cervical dilatations shown in Figure 4.4 confirms that almost half had it performed at or before 4 cm.

Regional analysis of these data gave small numbers only in each region. There was a trend for a higher rate of induction among the hospital booked/hospital delivered in Wales and Scotland. Similar trends were repeated in those who had an artificial rupture of membranes in labour for augmentation.

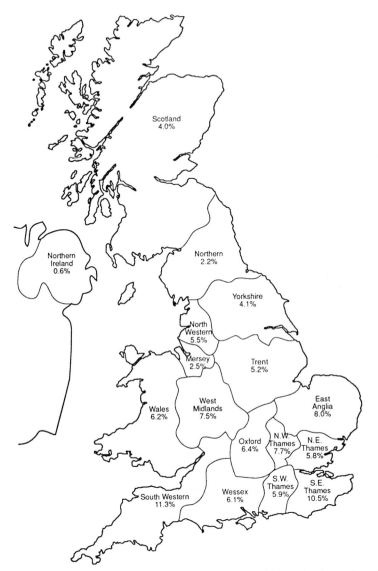

Figure 4.1 The regional distribution of births planned and delivered at home (NBTF Home Births Survey 1994)

LENGTH OF LABOUR

The length of labour is usually taken from when the woman first feels regular painful contractions until the delivery of the placenta and membranes. Conventionally it is divided into three stages:

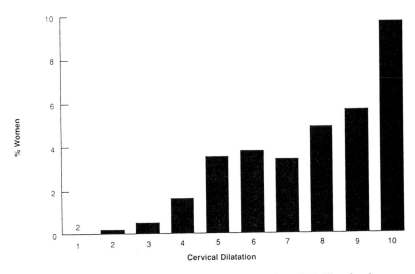

Figure 4.2 Artificial rupture of membrane by stage of cervical dilatation in women who had planned and delivered at home (NBTF Home Births Survey 1994)

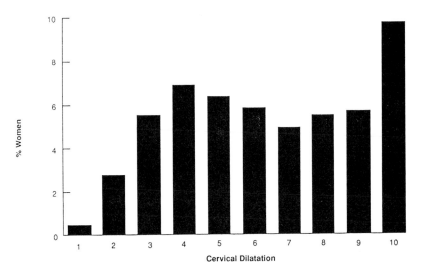

Figure 4.3 Artificial rupture of membrane by stage of cervical dilatation in women who had planned and delivered in hospital (NBTF Home Births Survey 1994)

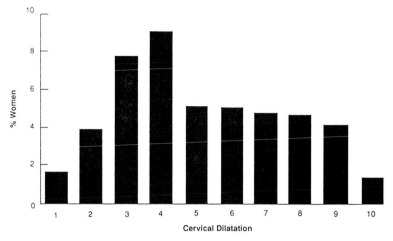

Figure 4.4 Artificial rupture of membrane by stage of cervical dilatation in women who planned home birth but delivered in hospital (NBTF Home Births Survey 1994)

Stage I   from the onset of labour to full dilatation of cervix;

Stage II   from full dilatation of cervix to delivery of the baby; and

Stage III from delivery of the baby to delivery of the placenta and membranes.

These stages are disparate, the first being very much longer than the second which in turn is usually longer than the third; the shortness of stage III is accentuated if assistance is given by an oxytocic agent at the end of stage II to hasten the delivery of the placenta.

Despite the inexactitudes of timing, these phases are commonly used maternity data and midwives are well used to this method of measurement. We asked date and time of the beginning of each stage and the end of the third stage so we could calculate the length of the first, second and third stages of labour.

Table 4.2 and Figure 4.5 show the data we received for first stage of labour.

The first two columns of Table 4.2 show those who delivered in the locus they had planned. The distribution over the time scale is virtually the same and there is no significant increase in the number of women who took more than 13 h in either case (6.9% and 6.7% respectively). However, among those who were home booked/hospital delivered it is very different ($p<0.0001$). There are fewer women in the under 12 h group and 29% who took more than 13 h, a figure over four times that found in those who delivered in the site they had chosen.

Table 4.2 Length of the first stage of labour reported by midwives (NBTF Home Births Survey 1994)

Length of first stage of labour (hours)	Planned and delivered at home (n = 3922)		Planned and delivered in hospital (n = 3319)		Planned home birth but delivered in hospital (n = 769)	
	n	%	n	%	n	%
<1	108	2.8	79	2.5	21	3.2
1–5	1817	47.7	1540	49.1	211	31.8
6–12	1624	42.6	1305	41.6	240	36.2
13–24	238	6.3	192	6.1	155	23.4
>24	21	0.6	18	0.6	36	5.4
Not known/ recorded	114		185		106	

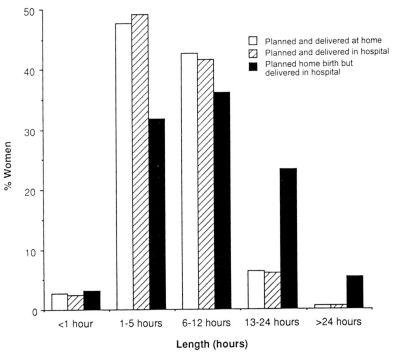

Figure 4.5 Length of the first stage of labour (NBTF Home Births Survey 1994)

Table 4.3 Length of the second stage of labour reported by midwives (NBTF Home Births Survey 1994)

Length of second stage of labour (minutes)	Planned and delivered at home (n = 3922)		Planned and delivered in hospital (n = 3319)		Planned home birth but delivered in hospital (n = 769)	
	n	%	n	%	n	%
<10	1432	37.5	1117	35.6	204	31.0
10–30	1530	40.1	1179	37.6	163	24.8
31–60	540	14.1	438	14	88	13.4
61–120	242	6.3	241	7.7	75	11.4
121–240	67	1.8	142	4.5	96	14.6
>240	6	0.2	22	0.7	32	4.9
Not known/ recorded	105		180		111	

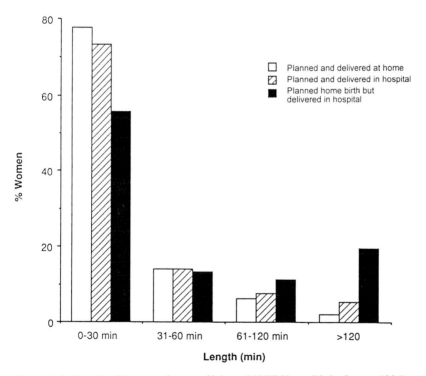

Figure 4.6 Length of the second stage of labour (NBTF Home Births Survey 1994)

A subset analysis was performed on the primigravid women who had planned a home delivery (790); of these 287 delivered in hospital. The proportion of these women who took more than 13 h in the first stage of labour is 31%; 89 of the 191 taking as long as this were primigravid. Table 4.3 and Figure 4.6 show the same data for the second stage of labour.

The second stage shows slight differences between the two groups who delivered where planned. The vast majority delivered inside an hour (92% and 87%) and indeed three-quarters of each group had delivered within 30 min in the second stage of labour. Whilst among those delivering at home 8% took over an hour, in the hospital group this was 13%, a significant difference ($p < 0.0001$). Comparing these women with those who transferred from home to hospital is also informative for 31% of the last group took over an hour in the second stage of labour. This is an almost quadrupling over those in the group home booked/home delivered and over doubling the hospital planned/hospital delivered. Again among the primigravidae who planned to deliver at home and took over an hour in the second stage, two-thirds of these delivered in hospital making up over half of the total transferred group (51%).

This is a study of those who had planned and had been accepted for home delivery, and so the total proportions of primigravidae are much lower than they would be in a total population of the UK (only 16% compared with over 39%). The rate of forceps deliveries in this group (7%) is not much greater than that of 5% in those who were hospital planned/hospital delivered. A possible reason for the long second stage could be that some were transferred in the second stage of labour which itself took time.

Table 4.4 and Figure 4.7 show the length of the third stage of labour; those who were home planned/home delivered reported a smaller proportion of placental delivery inside 10 min (62%) compared with the hospital group, (85%). The latter was very close to the group who were home planned/hospital delivered at 80%. There is a considerable increase in those taking half an hour to 3 h (10% of those at home births compared with 3% and 4% in the hospital delivered group). This may reflect the management of the third stage of labour of those at home; 56% at home had controlled cord traction compared with 86% and 69% in the other two groups respectively.

The giving of oxytocic drugs at the end of the second stage differed. Only 41% of those home planned/home delivered had syntometrine or ergometrine while 1% had syntocinon. Comparative figures for the other two groups were 53% and 7% and 43% and 12% respectively. The low

Table 4.4 Length of the third stage of labour reported by midwives (NBTF Home Births Survey 1994)

Length of third stage of labour (minutes)	Planned and delivered at home (*n* = 3896)		Planned and delivered in hospital (*n* = 3319)		Planned home birth but delivered in hospital (*n* = 769)	
	n	%	*n*	%	*n*	%
<5	1344	35.2	1680	53.4	348	52.3
5–10	1032	27.0	1001	31.8	182	27.3
11–30	1037	27.2	366	11.6	108	16.2
31–60	291	7.6	37	1.2	16	2.4
61–180	96	2.5	54	1.7	10	1.5
>180	16	0.4	8	0.3	2	0.3
Not known/ recorded	80		173		103	

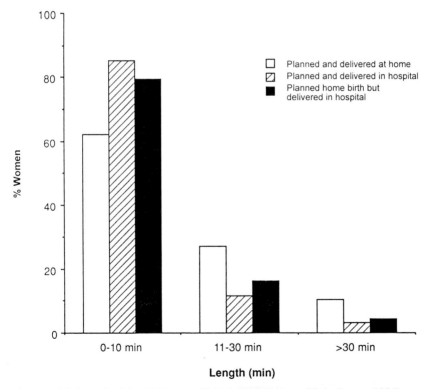

Figure 4.7 Length of the third stage of labour (NBTF Home Births Survey 1994)

rate of use of any oxytocic in the second stage in hospital and the even lower rate at home is disappointing given the strength of the evidence that routine use of oxytocics in the third stage of labour reduces the risk of postpartum haemorrhage by about 60%[1]. Midwives had been actively involved in many of the randomized trials that contributed to this evidence[2,3].

EATING AND DRINKING IN LABOUR

Questions were asked of all women concerning their wishes about drinking and eating during labour. Table 4.5 and Figure 4.8 show some of the responses from both the home planned/home delivered and those planning for hospital and giving birth in hospital.

Over 80% wished to drink during labour, mostly in early and mid-labour amongst the home deliveries. In actuality, three-quarters of the women drank in early and middle labour and a half in late labour. A similar breakdown is available for women in the hospital group which showed 63% to be drinking in early labour and 44% in late labour. In this group enquiries were made about the reasons given for women not being able to drink in labour; of the 259 women who reported a reason, almost a third (73) were told that it was against hospital policy and 70 that they may need a general anaesthetic. In 51 cases the woman was not given a reason.

The wish to eat in labour was much less strong; only a third (34%) of those delivering at home wished to eat in labour and 21% of the hospital group were similarly inclined. In actuality, in the home planned/home delivered group 90% ate in early labour, 35% in middle and 5% in late labour. In the hospital a lesser proportion of women wished to eat in labour. In this hospital group most of those who ate were in early labour with few in mid or late labour. Again 262 replies were received to questions about the reasons for being told they could not eat; 102 of these indicated that the woman may require a general anaesthetic and in 51 it was hospital policy not to allow this. In 42 instances there was no reason given.

The fasting of women in labour has been introduced since the association between aspiration pneumonitis (Mendelson's syndrome) and general anaesthesia during labour was made 40 years ago. Because strongly acid gastric contents might reflux up the oesophagus during general anaesthesia and spill over into the lungs, women were starved and forbidden to drink in the hope of reducing this complication. However,

Table 4.5 Wishes and actuality of eating and drinking in labour reported by women (NBTF Home Births Survey 1994)

| | Planned and delivered at home | | Planned and delivered in hospital | |
	n	%	n	%
Wished to drink	3521	84.1	2868	82.7
Not known/recorded	(6)		(34)	
$p<0.0001$				
Drank in labour				
early	2730	77.5	1805	62.9
middle	2666	75.7	2044	71.2
late	1778	50.5	1275	44.4
Wished to eat	1416	33.8	718	20.7
Not known/recorded	(7)		(38)	
$p<0.0001$				
Ate in labour				
early	1270	89.7	623	86.7
middle	502	35.4	202	28.1
late	72	5.0	40	5.5
Total	4191		3470	

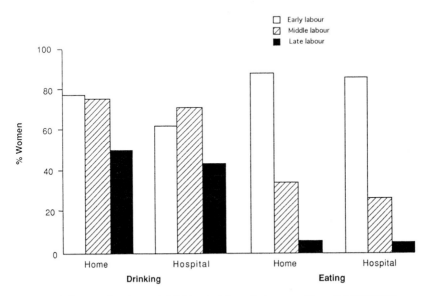

Figure 4.8 Reported eating and drinking in labour in home and hospital (NBTF Home Births Survey 1994)

gastric emptying itself is delayed in labour and this is increased by the giving of pethidine and opiate analgesia. Furthermore, food taken before going to hospital and additional gastric juice still being secreted would lodge in the stomach anyway.

Fewer women these days have a general anaesthetic as an emergency in labour. Rarely are forceps deliveries associated with general anaesthesia while many Caesarean sections are now performed under epidural or spinal anaesthesia. Pharmacological methods are available both to increase the rate of gastric emptying and to reduce the acidity in gastric contents. Among those who ate or drank in labour in our survey, very few had general anaesthetics. Between a half and a third of this subgroup who had Caesarean section seem to avoid general anaesthesia. In fact among the hospital planned/hospital delivered group only 2% of those who drank and ate also had a general anaesthetic.

Regional breakdown of answers to the questions by women did not show a great variation. Among those wishing to drink the range was 80% in Wales to 87% in South West Thames in the home planned/home delivered group. Comparable data in the hospital planned/hospital delivered group were very similar but a wider range is reported in the home planned/hospital delivered group: 75% in North Western region to 91% in Northern region.

Wanting to eat is reported less often and the regional ranges are rather wider, from 24% to 43% in the home planned/home delivered group, 5% to 26% in the hospital planned/hospital delivered group and 27% to 50% in the home planned/hospital delivered group. All these figures are small and no statistical significance tests were applied.

POSITION IN LABOUR

The position a woman adopts in labour should be that which she finds natural but usually is a consensus of two people's opinions – the woman and her professional attendant. In the last 100 years, it was often the professional who decided or even dictated the position a woman adopted. The doctors and many midwives preferred the woman to be on a firm bed for it was easier to guard and guide the passage of the baby over the perineum that way. Fifty years ago people used to lie flat on their backs or supine. That has not happened much in the last 30 years in the UK for it has been realized that when a heavily pregnant woman lies supine in late pregnancy, the uterus falls back on to the inferior vena cava so reducing blood return to the heart. A propped-up position with many pillows or the special National Childbirth Trust black rubber-covered wedge has been most commonly used for the last 30 years so that the woman is about 60° off the horizontal with her perineum close to the bed to receive the baby. Some professionals preferred to assist delivery in the left lateral position. That was popular in the seventeenth, eighteenth and nineteenth centuries and is well described by Smelley and others (Chapter 1).

It must be stressed that these positions are for delivery not for all the hours of labour. Many midwives and obstetricians are in favour of the woman walking or sitting in a chair as she wishes during the first stage of labour.

The woman's own wishes were often more instinctive, going back to older days described in Chapter 1. Women would squat or rest themselves kneeling on all fours; these ideas were handed down in families from a woman to her daughters. It is possible that the continued adoption of these positions has been a major factor which kept home births going, for community midwives have always been more sympathetic to women using these positions than were the more regimented teams in hospitals. Results are shown in Table 4.6 and Figure 4.9.

The reports of these were almost complete in the home planned/home delivered and hospital planned/hospital delivered women (columns 1 and 2 in Table 4.6); they were much less full from those who booked at home and gave birth in hospital (3% missing data). Using the information provided in Table 4.6, it would seem that 50% of women who were home planned/home delivered (column 1 in Table 4.6) had delivered off the bed compared with 14% of the hospital planned/hospital delivered. The commonest not-in-bed position adopted was on all fours reported by 886 women (23% of the 3896 women giving birth at home) with variations of this in kneeling and squatting making up 14%. Some 279 women (7%) adopted a sitting position of an unspecified nature and 20 more women reported using a birth chair or cushion. This may have reflected the absence of available birth chairs in the home rather than the lack of wish to use one.

The standing position was reported by 209 women (5%); this is a traditional position used in many non-European countries particularly in Africa.

The use of waterbirths in the home was examined; we asked a specific question about birth taking place in water to which 156 women (4%) who were home planned/home delivered answered yes but only 1% in the hospital planned/hospital delivered group.

Table 4.6 Positions reported by midwives for women delivering in booked place of delivery and those transferred to hospital after home booking (NBTF Home Births Survey 1994)

	Planned and delivered at home		Planned and delivered in hospital		Planned home birth but delivered in hospital	
	n	*%*	*n*	*%*	*n*	*%*
In bed						
Propped up	1527	38.8	2147	64.7	310	40.3
Lateral and lateral tilt	324	8.3	383	11.5	131	17.0
Supine	62	1.6	107	3.2	43	5.6
Lithotomy	1	—	194	5.8	122	15.9
Subtotal	1914	48.7	2831	85.2	606	78.8
Not in bed						
Sitting	279	7.2	223	6.7	35	4.6
Sitting in birth chair or on cushion	20	0.4	12	0.4	8	1.0
Standing	209	5.4	28	0.9	11	1.4
Squatting	310	8.0	20	0.6	19	2.5
Kneeling	229	5.9	28	0.9	12	1.5
All fours	886	22.4	143	4.3	50	6.5
Floating (in water birth)	19	0.5	8	0.3	2	0.3
Subtotal	1951	49.8	462	13.9	137	17.8
Not known/ not recorded	57	1.5	26	0.8	26	3.4
Total	3922	100.0	3319	99.9	769	100.0

The remaining women in this group included 1527 (39%) who delivered in a propped-up position and 324 (8%) who reported use of a lateral or lateral tilt position. Only 62 women (2%) were supine and one woman was in a lithotomy position though there are no details as to how she was able to maintain this in the home with an absence of lithotomy poles.

One mother who gave birth at home, having already experienced two hospital births, had this to say:

> It is very sad that most hospitals are interventionist and so clinical in their labour wards, and that ultimately most women find themselves on their backs giving birth, the worst possible position to be in – all for the midwives' convenience.

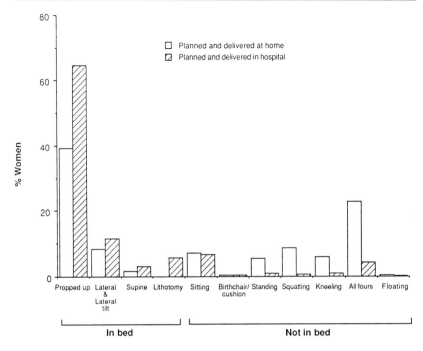

Figure 4.9 Positions reported for women delivering in booked place of delivery (NBTF Home Births Survey 1994)

The middle column of Table 4.6 examines those 3319 women who were hospital planned/hospital delivered. The positions used are in entirely different proportions; here, 85% of them delivered on a bed, almost 65% were propped up and 12% in a lateral position; the supine position was used by 3% and lithotomy in 194 (6%). This last may well have been associated with a forceps delivery or vacuum extraction.

Some 462 only of these women (14%), adopted positions that were not on the bed; of these 223 (7%) were sitting with 12 women reported using a birth chair or cushion. This is a disappointingly small number considering the large outlay on birth chairs and cushions. In the 1984 National Birthday Trust Fund (NBTF) Survey on Facilities Available at the Place of Birth, 18% of delivery units had a birth chair so that by extrapolation of birth numbers, 28% of women delivering had access to one. A cluster of higher frequency was shown then in the Yorkshire, Mersey and North Western Regional Health Authorities where 47% of women respectively had access compared with Oxford which reported only 2% of women were so provided[4]. We have no national data since then for a decade and so cannot comment precisely but this seems an under use of potentially useful equipment.

Twenty-eight women reported standing; squatting, kneeling and on all fours was used by 6% compared with 37% of the home planned/home delivered group of women. Thirty-three women (1%) were reported to have water births and 266 (8%) used warm water in the first stage of labour; this may reflect a more regimental approach towards women who go to hospital.

One mother included the following in a list of things she did not like about the birth in hospital:

> ...not allowed to get into positions comfortable for you. They had to be easy for the midwife ... not asked about positions before second stage, birth chair or pool.

Among the 769 women who had booked for home delivery but were transferred to hospital in late pregnancy or in labour the positions show a mixed picture (Table 4.6, column 3). Some 606 women (79%) delivered on the bed while 18% did not use this facility. These are much closer to the proportions in the hospital planned/hospital delivered group than in the home planned/home delivered group. The propped-up position was used in 40%, virtually the same proportion as the home planned/home delivered group, but the lateral position was increased in use significantly over both the other groups. Supine position was used in 6% and lithotomy in 16%, a probable indication of the increased use of operative vaginal deliveries for this group of women had a high proportion of forceps and vacuum operative deliveries (17%).

Tables 4.7 and 4.8 with Figures 4.10 to 4.13 show the regional analysis of these data. Numbers are small in some regions; Figure 4.13 shows insignificant trends in the lesser use of the all fours position in the Northern and Western regions of the country. The analysis of the hospital planned/hospital delivered group (Table 4.8) have few data in each box but is included for comparison.

The squatting and kneeling positions were generally most popularly used; it is probable that these positions give the woman most satisfaction and may even relieve some of the discomfort of labour. Professionals should listen more to women and help them adopt positions in labour that they instinctively wish to take up. Provided women are not putting themselves or their fetuses in danger, professional stances should change; the new ideas are really the old ones from ancient Egypt referred to in Chapter 1. Perhaps the birth chair is rejected for ill-understood reasons but

Table 4.7 Regional analysis of position used in delivery in the home planned/home delivered group reported by midwives (NBTF Home Births Survey 1994)

Region	In bed n	In bed %	All fours n	All fours %	Sitting n	Sitting %	Standing n	Standing %	Squatting n	Squatting %	Other n	Other %
Northern	46	56.8	18	22.2	9	11.1	2	2.5	3	3.7	3	3.7
Yorkshire	88	60.6	26	17.9	16	11.0	7	4.8	4	2.8	4	2.8
Trent	113	62.0	30	16.5	16	8.8	4	2.2	11	6.0	6	3.3
East Anglia	143	49.3	68	23.4	19	6.6	17	5.9	22	7.6	21	7.2
North West Thames	96	36.9	67	25.8	23	8.8	19	7.3	40	15.4	12	4.6
North East Thames	71	38.1	53	27.3	9	4.6	14	7.2	23	11.9	19	9.8
South East Thames	148	43.0	87	23.8	18	4.9	24	6.6	31	8.5	47	12.9
South West Thames	70	34.0	59	28.6	16	7.8	15	7.3	21	10.2	25	12.1
Wessex	160	52.6	53	24.7	6	2.8	12	5.6	12	5.6	17	7.9
Oxford	105	45.1	57	24.5	26	11.2	13	5.6	15	6.4	17	7.3
South Western	171	43.6	120	30.5	23	5.9	20	5.1	36	9.2	22	5.6
West Midlands	148	57.8	60	23.4	14	5.5	12	4.7	14	5.5	7	2.7
Mersey	56	64.4	9	10.3	6	6.9	3	3.4	10	11.5	2	2.3
North Western	131	66.9	21	10.7	10	5.1	7	3.6	9	4.6	17	8.7
Northern Ireland	14	73.7	1	5.3	2	10.5	1	5.3	1	5.3	0	—
Scotland	59	38.4	40	26.5	14	9.3	12	7.9	12	7.9	15	9.9
Wales	134	61.6	36	16.5	21	9.6	11	5.0	1	5.3	1	0.5
Not known/ recorded 385												
Total	1753	50.0	805	23.0	248	7.0	193	5.5	265	7.9	235	6.6

Table 4.8 Regional analysis of position used in delivery in the hospital planned/ hospital delivered group reported by midwives (NBTF Home Births Survey 1994)

Region	In bed n	In bed %	All fours n	All fours %	Sitting n	Sitting %	Standing n	Standing %	Squatting n	Squatting %	Other n	Other %
Northern	78	83.8	3	3.2	11	11.8	1	1.1	0	—	0	—
Yorkshire	135	91.2	5	3.4	6	4.1	2	1.4	0	—	0	—
Trent	128	91.5	1	0.7	7	5.0	0	—	1	0.7	3	2.1
East Anglia	182	80.6	17	7.5	17	16.6	5	2.2	0	—	6	2.7
North West Thames	140	80.0	9	5.1	15	8.6	4	2.3	3	1.7	4	2.3
North East Thames	87	85.3	6	5.9	7	6.9	1	1.0	1	1.0	0	—
South East Thames	150	84.8	8	4.5	6	3.4	4	2.3	4	2.3	4	2.3
South West Thames	106	87.6	6	5.0	6	5.0	1	0.8	0	—	1	0.8
Wessex	109	90.0	2	1.7	7	5.8	0	—	1	0.8	2	1.7
Oxford	145	78.8	16	8.7	15	8.2	2	1.1	0	—	6	3.3
South Western	270	80.4	25	7.6	26	8.0	3	0.9	4	1.2	5	1.5
West Midlands	184	88.4	5	2.4	15	7.2	2	1.0	1	0.5	0	—
Mersey	44	84.5	4	7.7	3	5.8	0	—	1	1.9	0	—
North Western	134	94.3	3	2.1	4	2.8	0	—	0	—	1	0.7
Northern Ireland	19	100.0	0	—	0	—	0	—	0	—	0	—
Scotland	154	87.6	3	1.7	18	10.2	0	—	0	—	1	0.6
Wales	164	89.6	7	3.8	9	4.2	0	—	1	0.5	0	—
Not known/ recorded	725											
Total	2229	86.0	120	4.6	170	6.5	25	0.9	17	0.6	33	1.2

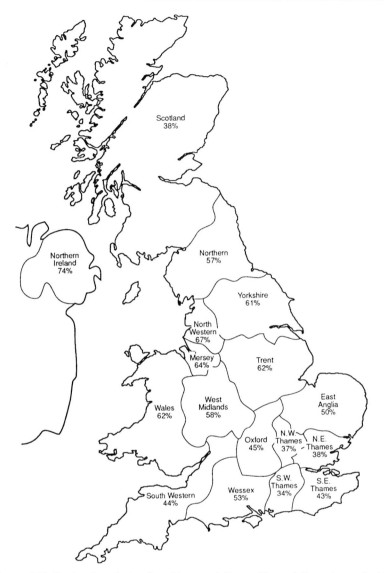

Figure 4.10 Regional analysis of positions at delivery. Those delivered on a bed in the home booked/home delivered group – see Table 4.7 column 1 (NBTF Home Births Survey 1994)

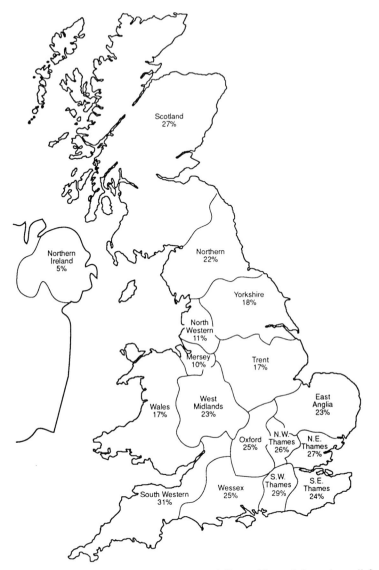

Figure 4.11 Regional analysis of positions at delivery. Those delivered on all fours in the home booked/home delivered group (NBTF Home Births Survey 1994)

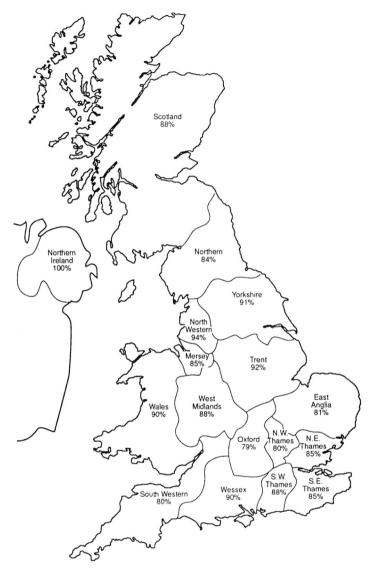

Figure 4.12 Regional analysis of positions at delivery. Those delivered on a bed in the hospital booked/home delivered group – see Table 4.8, column 1 (NBTF Home Births Survey 1994)

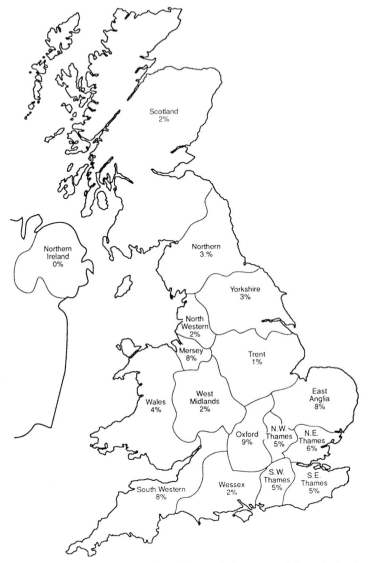

Figure 4.13 Regional analysis of positions at delivery on all fours in the hospital booked/hospital delivered group – see Table 4.8 column 2 (NBTF Home Births Survey 1994)

it is the women having the babies who should choose, not a group of interested lay people nor professional attendants.

METHOD OF DELIVERY

Most women deliver naturally. We anticipated a particularly high rate of spontaneous vaginal delivery among the low-risk women recruited to this study. Tables 4.9 and 4.10 with Figure 4.14 show how women who intended to deliver at home had a significantly higher rate of spontaneous vaginal delivery (94.1%) than women who intended to deliver in hospital (90%). The differences in the rate of assisted vaginal delivery and Caesarean section seen between the two groups may be due in part to the limitations of the matching process described in Chapter 3. It seems likely however that some of the differences in intervention rates must be due to the intended place of birth. The reasons for the variation in intervention rates between two populations of similar obstetric risk are complex. The hypothesis that social and environmental factors can affect progress of labour and mode of delivery is strongly supported by experimental evidence. A systematic review of randomized controlled trials shows that continuous professional support during labour is associated with a reduced incidence of Caesarean section and instrumental delivery[5]. In the light of this evidence it is easy to accept that some women may labour better in their own homes.

The most common indications for obstetric intervention, dystocia and fetal distress, are both based on soft diagnostic criteria[6]. Enormous variations in the rates at which these conditions are diagnosed have been observed between and within obstetric institutions throughout the world. It is inevitable that differences in these diagnoses would occur between midwives caring for women at home and midwives and doctors caring for women in hospital. At the risk of stating the obvious, a final explanation for the variation in the rate of operative delivery is the fact that the opportunity for assisted delivery is abolished by home birth. No Caesarean section or instrumental delivery took place at home and in some cases transfer from home to hospital took place because of a perceived need for intervention delivery.

Table 4.9 Methods of delivery by place of intent at 37 weeks reported by midwives (NBTF Home Births Survey 1994)

	Booked for home delivery (n = 4705)		*Booked for hospital delivery* (n = 3352)	
	n	*%*	*n*	*%*
Spontaneous				
cephalic	4390	94.1	3005	89.6
other	30	0.6	20	0.6
p<0.0001				
Assisted				
vaginal	115	2.4	180	5.4
Caesarean section	94	2.0	139	4.1
Not known/recorded	76		8	

Spontaneous cephalic includes OA, occipito-anterior; OT, occipito-transverse; OP, occipito-posterior
Spontaneous other include Breech, Face and Compound
Assisted vaginal includes Forceps and Vacuum extraction

Table 4.10 Methods of delivery by actual place of birth reported by midwives (NBTF Home Births Survey 1994)

	Planned and delivered at home (n = 3922)		*Planned and delivered in hospital* (n = 3319)		*Planned home birth but delivered in hospital* (n = 769)		*Planned hospital birth but delivered at home* (n = 33)	
	n	*%*	*n*	*%*	*n*	*%*	*n*	*%*
Spontaneous								
cephalic	3855	98.2	2974	89.8	535	69.6	31	100
other	16	0.4	20	0.8	14	1.8	0	—
p<0.0001								
Assisted								
vaginal	0	—	180	5.4	115	16.9	0	—
Caesarean section	0	—	139	4.2	94	15.0	0	—
Not known/ recorded	51		6		11		2	

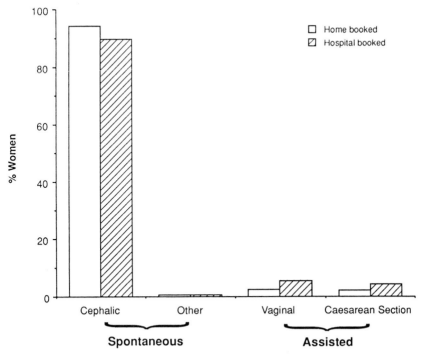

Figure 4.14 Methods of delivery by place of booking (NBTF Home Births Survey 1994)

Among the 3915 multiparous women who had booked and been accepted for a home delivery, 381 (9.7%) had a previous operative vaginal delivery and 53 (1.4%) had a previous Caesarean section. In this subset with an operative delivery in the past, 59 (15.6%) of those who had had a forceps or vacuum extraction, were transferred for hospital delivery compared with 11% of the whole multiparous group. Fifteen of the 53 who had a Caesarean section before were also transferred, 28% of this group indicating the increased anxiety in the minds of the professionals about a Caesarean section in a previous pregnancy.

Tables 4.11 and 4.12 (and Figures 4.15 and 4.16) relate to the regional breakdown of methods of delivery of the groups by planning intent. In all regions the home-booked group achieved a spontaneous cephalic delivery in over 90% (99% in Mersey). The lower rates in Northern region and Scotland (90% and 91%) are concomitant with much higher proportion of Caesarean section (8% and 5% respectively).

The sample is large enough and may reflect a population of women who tend to produce a greater number of late pregnancy or labour

Table 4.11 Regional analysis of method of delivery of women booked for home delivery reported by midwives (NBTF Home Births Survey 1994)

| | Spontaneous | | | | Assisted | | | |
| | Cephalic | | Other | | Vaginal | | Caesarean section | |
Region	n	%	n	%	n	%	n	%
Northern	110	90.2	1	0.8	1	0.8	10	8.2
Yorkshire	195	95.1	2	1.0	4	2.0	3	1.5
Trent	227	94.6	0	—	6	2.5	7	2.9
East Anglia	348	96.9	0	—	8	2.2	2	0.6
North West Thames	334	93.1	3	0.9	12	3.3	10	2.8
North East Thames	254	94.4	1	0.4	8	2.9	4	1.5
South East Thames	454	94.2	2	0.4	12	2.5	12	2.5
South West Thames	263	93.2	4	1.4	8	2.9	5	1.8
Wessex	259	95.2	1	0.4	6	2.2	6	2.2
Oxford	285	95.3	2	0.7	9	3.0	2	0.7
South Western	499	96.7	4	0.8	15	2.9	11	2.1
West Midlands	337	95.5	5	1.4	8	2.2	2	0.6
Mersey	106	99.1	0	—	0	—	1	0.9
North Western	240	96.8	1	0.4	3	1.2	4	1.6
Northern Ireland	23	95.8	0	—	0	—	0	—
Scotland	197	91.2	0	—	9	4.2	10	4.6
Wales	273	95.8	0	—	6	1.4	4	1.4
Not known/ recorded 67								
Total	4404	95.0	26	0.5	115	2.5	93	2.0

complications or that this screening process for choosing women for home delivery may require re-examination in these regions. Alternatively, the obstetricians in these parts of the country may be more inclined to intervene. This hypothesis is borne out in Table 4.12 where the hospital-intended group of women also show higher Caesarean section rates.

The analysis of method of delivery is also performed from data in Table 4.10 which show reported results by the place of actual delivery. Columns 1 and 2 are the major groups of those who delivered where planned and show a similar picture to Table 4.9 about spontaneous cephalic deliveries being 99% for the former and 90% in the latter. However amongst those who were home booked/hospital delivered (some 769 women in column 3), only 70% had spontaneous cephalic delivery. Whilst the spontaneous breech, face and compound deliveries were slightly increased (although

Table 4.12 Regional analysis of method of delivery of women booked for hospital delivery reported by midwives (NBTF Home Births Survey 1994)

| | Spontaneous | | | | Assisted | | | |
| | Cephalic | | Other | | Vaginal | | Caesarean section | |
Region	n	%	n	%	n	%	n	%
Northern	104	91.3	0	—	3	2.6	7	6.1
Yorkshire	173	91.6	2	1.1	3	1.6	10	5.3
Trent	164	90.7	0	—	11	6.1	6	3.3
East Anglia	249	92.6	1	0.4	10	3.7	7	2.6
North West Thames	195	87.1	0	—	17	7.6	11	4.9
North East Thames	120	85.7	4	2.9	13	9.3	3	2.1
South East Thames	202	87.0	0	—	17	7.3	12	5.2
South West Thames	145	87.9	0	—	10	6.0	10	6.1
Wessex	147	87.5	2	1.2	10	6.0	9	5.4
Oxford	220	90.5	0	—	12	5.0	11	4.5
South Western	370	89.8	2	0.5	22	5.4	16	3.9
West Midlands	264	91.4	2	0.7	15	5.2	8	2.8
Mersey	56	87.5	0	—	6	9.4	2	3.1
North Western	177	89.8	2	1.0	12	6.1	6	3.0
Northern Ireland	23	95.8	0	—	1	4.2	0	—
Scotland	166	88.5	1	0.5	11	5.8	9	4.8
Wales	219	91.6	1	0.4	7	3.0	12	5.0
Not known/ recorded 22								
Total	2994	89.9	17	0.5	180	5.4	139	4.2

not significantly so over the other two major groups for numbers were small), this deficit in vaginal deliveries is mostly explained by the differences in assisted vaginal deliveries and Caesarean sections. In this group, the Northern region had the highest Caesarean section rate at 7% although numbers are not very large.

There were no vaginal assisted deliveries (forceps or vacuum extraction) in the home-reported births amongst the 3896 who delivered there. This reflects 1994 general practitioner obstetrics; those doctors who were used to applying forceps in the home have now retired. Amongst the hospital planned/hospital delivered women the forceps rate was 5%, about half the rate nationally and reflecting the method of choosing the hospital controls in this survey based on a population booked for home delivery. Those who were home planned/hospital delivered had a forceps rate of 17%. The need for an assisted delivery may have been the reason for the transfers in many cases.

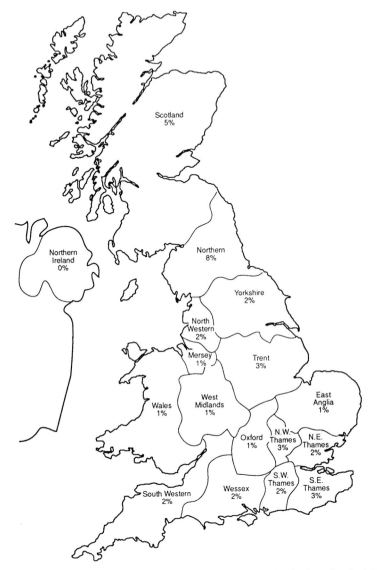

Figure 4.15 Regional analysis of proportion of Caesarean section in those booked for home delivery (NBTF Home Births Survey 1994)

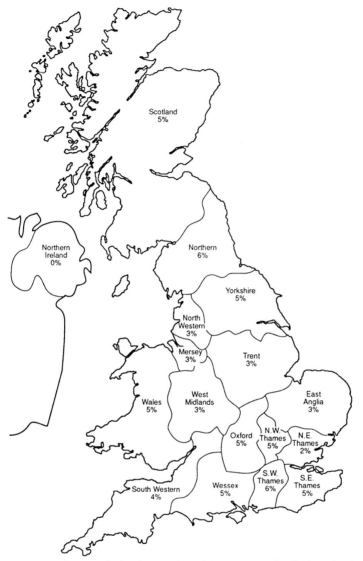

Figure 4.16 Regional analysis of proportion of Caesarean section in those booked for hospital delivery (NBTF Home Births Survey 1994)

Similar differences are shown with Caesarean section rates in Figures 4.15 and 4.16. Obviously none were in the home planned/home delivered group. The rate for the hospital planned/hospital delivered women was 4%, well below national data; imprecise though such statutory data now are, the Caesarean section rate was probably around 16% in 1994. The home planned/hospital delivered group had a Caesarean section rate of 15%, three times that of the hospital planned/hospital delivered group.

These increased rates of operative delivery in those home planned/ hospital delivered women are some indication of the staff and facilities implications which are required for those women that have to transfer. The reduction of staffing levels in the main hospitals because of any small shift into the domiciliary sector or isolated midwifery units would seem unwise with these data in mind.

WHO DELIVERS?

The answer to the simple question 'Who delivered a woman?' is not easy. If only one midwife was in the room the answer is clear. However, if there are two midwives one of whom is senior to the other, it is sometimes difficult to know which was the actual person although the questionnaire specifically did ask who actually did the delivery. The situation becomes more complex when there is a mixture of doctors and midwives in the room, particularly if they are of different seniorities. It might be claimed in law that the most senior obstetrical person present would be responsible and therefore was in charge of delivery although a medical student or junior midwife might have actually had hands on the perineum. The midwife, however, is still accountable for her own practice.

In our survey we looked at the answers to this question in several ways.

Table 4.13 shows the answer to the questions in the midwives' questionnaires for both home planned and hospital planned deliveries. The question (B13 and B14 respectively) asked who delivered the baby and they were asked to respond by ticking only one box. Of the 4705 women delivering at home 4699 people were ticked as being the sole person who delivered. In the hospital, for the 3352 women who had a baby, 3390 personnel were recorded as the sole person who delivered. In 38 cases more than one person was identified as having been the sole person who delivered the baby, e.g. student midwife and qualified midwife.

Among the home planned 93% were delivered by midwives, 5% by a doctor, 0.2% by other medically-associated personnel and 2% by someone

Table 4.13 Reported personnel who delivered the woman by their place of intended delivery reported by midwives (NBTF Home Births Survey 1994)

	Home planned		Hospital planned	
Midwives				
Grade E	186		1006	
F	293		494	
G	3338		1000	
H	98		44	
I	16		6	
Other midwife	4		8	
Independent	221		4	
Student	230		394	
Total midwives	4386	(92.7%)	2956	(86.9%)
*Doctors**				
SHO	23		52	
Registrar	128		223	
Senior registrar	56		51	
Consultant	14		18	
GP	23		3	
Total doctors	244	(5.2%)	347	(10.2%)
Other medically associated				
Medical student	5		75	
Other student	0		0	
Nurse (not midwife)	2		3	
Ambulance officer	1		1	
Total other medically associated	8	(0.2%)	79	(2.3%)
Other				
Family or friend	53		7	
No one	8		1	
Not known/ not recorded	30		11	
Total other	91	(1.9%)	19	(0.6%)
Total	4729		3401	

*SHO, Senior house officer; GP, general practitioner

in the other group including 53 women delivered by family or a friend and eight where the midwife reported there was no one present.

Comparing these with the women who were planned for a hospital delivery, almost 6% less were delivered by a midwife (87%) with almost twice the number of doctors delivering (10%). A large part of the increase in the other medically-associated deliverers was made up of medical students and nurses who were not midwives. There was perhaps some confusion in the mind of those who filled in the form for they might have coded them as nurses rather than student midwives. Fewer family or friends performed delivery in hospital (seven compared with 53) and only one woman was reported to be alone in the hospital planned group compared with eight in the domiciliary booked.

Among the midwives taking part in deliveries there was a distinct difference in seniority among those who looked after women with a planned home birth and those with a planned hospital birth. In the home intended group there were 4156 women delivered by a trained midwife (excluding the 230 student midwife deliveries). Of these some 80% were delivered by a G grade midwife, 11% had someone more junior than this and 3% had a more senior midwife. The remaining 5% were independent midwives whose posts are not graded. Seniority will be considered further when we examine the lead professional in each instance. Similar data for the hospital booked women showed a G grade midwife as deliverer in 39%, about half the proportion in the home deliveries. Junior midwives made up 58%, over five times that of the home deliveries, while more senior grades delivered 2%. Independent midwives performed 221 deliveries in the home but only four in the hospital planned group.

Further analysis was made of the deliveries by both intent and actual place where the women did deliver (Table 4.14). The proportions are the same order but it will be seen that over 97% of all of deliveries in the home planned/home delivered group were by midwives compared with 1% by general practitioners or their trainees. In the hospital planned/hospital delivered group the midwives still performed 87% of deliveries with 10% being performed by doctors. Among this medically-delivered group only 15% (52 cases) were delivered by senior house officers. This is how it should be, for if a case is outside the limits of midwifery practice, then a more experienced obstetrician than a senior house officer should take over. Excluding the three delivered by general practitioners, the rest were all performed by registrars, senior registrars, or consultants. Medical students performed 75 of the deliveries under the supervision of a trained midwife or doctor.

Among those in the home planned/hospital delivered group, 68% had a midwife; almost 30% were delivered by doctors, again with a heavy trend towards using more experienced doctors. Medical students still took part in five of these deliveries.

Table 4.14 Reported personnel who delivered women by their place of intent and where they actually delivered reported by midwives (NBTF Home Births Survey 1994)

	Planned and delivered at home		Planned and delivered in hospital		Planned home birth but delivered in hospital		Planned hospital birth but delivered at home		Total
Midwives									
Grade E	61		1006		124		0		1191
F	226		493		62		1		782
G	3032		978		282		22		4314
H	91		43		7		1		142
I	15		6		0		0		21
Other midwife	4		8		0		0		12
Independent	200		3		18		1		222
Student	191		392		38		2		623
Total midwives	3820	(97.6%)	2929	(87%)	531	(67.8%)	27	(79.4%)	
*Doctors**									
SHO	0		52		23		0		75
Registrar	0		223		128		0		351
Senior registrar	0		51		56		0		107
Consultant	0		18		14		0		32
GP	18		3		3		0		24
Total doctors	18	(0.5%)	347	(10.2%)	224	(28.6%)	0		
Others medically associated									
Medical student	0		75		5		0		80
Nurse (not midwife)	0		3		1		0		4
Ambulance officer	0		0		0		1		1
Total other medical	0		78	(2.3%)	6	(0.8%)	1	(2.9%)	
Others									
Family or friend	54		1		0		6		61
No one	7		0		0		0		7
Not known/ not recorded	23		11		22		0		38
Total others	84	(2.1%)	12	(0.4%)	22	(2.8%)	6	(17.7%)	
Total	3922		3366		783		34		

*SHO, senior house officer; GP, general practitioner

In the very small group of 33 women who were hospital planned/home delivered 79% were delivered by a midwife of whom the vast majority were G grade. One was delivered by an ambulance officer.

Again in Table 4.14 we analysed the grade of the midwife who delivered. Of those whose grades were known in the home planned/home delivered group 78% were G Grade, 8% being junior and 3% being more senior. This proportion dropped in the hospital planned/hospital delivered group where only 34% were G Grade with 54% being junior and only 2% being senior. Among the group of those who were home planned/hospital delivered 50% were delivered by G Grade midwives, 35% by junior and 1% by more senior midwives. For completeness, in the hospital planned/home delivered group 22 were G Grade midwives with one other being senior and three being more junior.

The independent midwives were again working mostly in the home planned group; 200 of them delivered the home planned/home delivered group and 18 independent midwives went into the hospital with the home planned/hospital delivered women to deliver their charge there. Of the 3308 women who were hospital planned/hospital delivered, only three were delivered by independent midwives and one independent midwife looked after a women who was hospital planned/home delivered; thus were 222 deliveries cared for by independent midwives.

Student midwives were described as the deliverer in 623 cases; trained midwives in E Grade delivered 1191 and F Grade 782 but the vast majority were G Grade who delivered 4314 women. More senior midwives made up 163 deliverers only.

In this survey the hospital doctors did not deliver anyone outside the hospital; inside it was mostly the senior doctors who acted with only 75 senior house officers performing deliveries. Family or a friend delivered the woman in 61 instances of which only one was in the hospital. On eight occasions in the home planned/home delivered group the woman was reported as having nobody with her.

Because of the problems of deciding who actually delivered we asked about the *lead professional* at the delivery. This person might not have been the actual assistant but would have been supervising the birth. This new phrase stems from *Changing Childbirth* where the Department of Health wished to nominate a non-statutory title for the professional to whom the woman could turn in pregnancy and who was to be responsible for ensuring the other professionals in the team were involved at the right times through antenatal care and delivery. The concept probably is more useful in antenatal care than labour but it is a term being bandied around widely and therefore the National Birthday Trust Fund survey team thought it would be as another pointer to whom the midwives thought was in charge of the delivery.

Table 4.15 shows the reported data for those women planning a home delivery or a hospital delivery.

It is seen that in the home planned group 95% had a midwife as the lead professional and 5% a doctor. Of the midwives 87% were G grade, 11%

Table 4.15 The lead professional at normal delivery reported by midwives (NBTF Home Births Survey 1994)

	Home planned		Hospital planned	
Midwife				
Grade E	137		1027	
F	265		568	
G	3448		1182	
H	114		53	
I	16		10	
Other midwife				
Independent	224		2	
Student	2		7	
Total midwives	4206	(95.3%)	2849	(94.7%)
*Doctor**				
SHO	5		20	
Registrar	85		61	
Senior Registrar	52		46	
Consultant	14		24	
GP	38		8	
Other doctor				
Total doctors	194	(4.7%)	159	(5.3%)
Not known/reported	531		344	
Total reported	4400		3008	

*SHO, senior house officer; GP, general practitioner

below it and 4% more senior. Compared with this, in the hospital planned group, 95% midwives also were noted as the lead professional in labour, with a doctor as the lead professional in 5%, no significant difference from the home planned group. However, breaking down the grade of midwife showed that only 42% were G grade with 56% junior to this; 2% were senior. This shows the different usage of midwives in the hospital where a much more junior midwife, commonly grade E, is used to be the lead professional at delivery presumably with other more senior midwives available if need arises.

Some women, who chose to have their babies at home, were reported by the midwives as a cause for concern when advice was ignored. Examples given were: refusing to be transferred to hospital when problems arose; refusing to allow the midwife to listen to the baby's heart beat; insisting on giving birth to the baby in water although advised to use the water only for pain relief. Such instances can put a heavy responsibility on to the shoulders of the midwife. The support of another more experienced midwife within the same team or the Supervisor of Midwives on call was reported to be available and appreciated.

In 38 instances of home planned and home delivered women, the GP was reported as the lead professional (1%). Otherwise the involvement of the doctor as lead professional in the home planned deliveries comes entirely from the group who were transferred from home to hospital in late pregnancy or early labour, for no hospital doctors were involved with delivery in the home. Again this shows that if the woman is transferred with some problem it is the registrar/senior registrar who takes the lead in most cases (72% of instances).

The use of the independent midwives as a lead professional was almost entirely confined to those with home planned deliveries. However, when some women had to be transferred from their planned home delivery to the hospital, the independent midwife often went also and as Table 4.15 shows was the lead professional inside the hospital as well. This is as it should be if a lead professional is going to give continuity of care.

The term lead professional is a new one and is not precise in the minds of many midwives and doctors or even in the Department of Health. This is reflected in the student midwives and senior house officers being designated lead professional when it is extremely unlikely that they really were. The term lead professional and the person who delivers has been confused.

PAIN RELIEF IN LABOUR

The methods of pain relief used in 8676 instances for home booked and 5953 occasions for the hospital booked women are recorded. Since there were 4489 and 3165 women respectively who answered this question in these groups, many must have tried more than one method, the rates of reported usage being ×1.9 and ×1.4 per woman respectively. The actual numbers of methods used per woman is probably greater than this; 798 and 287 women respectively were reported as having no analgesia while a small number of other methods was employed (Table 4.16 and Figure 4.17).

Generally the use of pharmacological methods was much lower in the home booked compared with the hospital booked. One mother remarked:

> I am sure that the very relaxing atmosphere caused by being at home was the reason I was able to give birth using only breathing exercises for pain relief.

Table 4.16 The analgesia used by 4705 women who had planned a home birth and 3352 planning a hospital birth reported by midwives. More than one method was often used by one woman so totals are >100% (NBTF Home Births Survey 1994)

	Planned home delivery (*n* = 8676)		*Planned hospital delivery* (*n* = 5953)	
	n	%	*n*	%
Pharmacological methods				
Nitrous oxide	2464	52.6	2409	72.1
$p < 0.0001$				
Pethidine	350	7.5	1013	30.3
$p < 0.0001$				
Epidural	137	2.8	377	11.3
$p < 0.0001$				
Spinal	33	0.7	42	1.3
$p = 0.0068$				
Non-pharmacological methods				
$p < 0.0001$				
Relaxation	2291	49.0	1004	30.1
TENS*	1030	22.0	515	15.4
Warm water	1143	24.4	267	8.0
Aromatherapy	243	5.2	29	0.9
Homeopathy	159	3.4	9	0.3
Acupuncture	28	0.6	1	—
None	798	17.1	287	8.6
Not known/recorded	216		187	

*TENS, transcutaneous electrical nerve stimulation

It was notable that only 8% of women with planned home births used pethidine (compared with 30% in hospital). The comparative portability of this drug obviously could not make up for the perceived loss of control of labour by the mother and the worries of the midwife about neonatal respiratory depression. Nitrous oxide premixed with oxygen (Entonox) was used by a half planning home births and three-quarters of the hospital group.

Non-pharmacological methods were much more used by the home booked, almost half using relaxation techniques (cf. 30% hospital booked) and 24% using warm water (8% in hospital). Transcutaneous electrical nerve stimulation (TENS) was employed by 22% and 15% respectively while aromatherapy, homeopathy and acupuncture were used by a few at home and fewer in the hospital groups. Satisfaction was harder to assess for it meant comparing the midwives' reports of analgesia actually used with the woman's answers and the denominators were different.

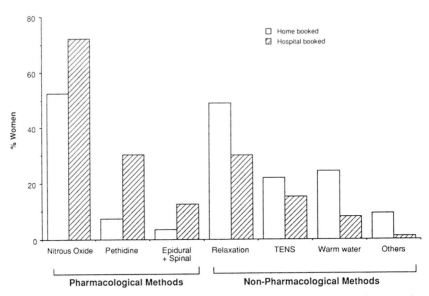

Figure 4.17 The analgesia used by place of booking. More than one method was used sometimes by one woman (NBTF Home Births Survey 1994)

It was obvious that some of the analgesia methods used by women booked for home delivery would not have been used in the domestic scene, e.g. epidural and spinal anaesthesia. The data were therefore reanalysed by actual place of birth as laid down earlier in this chapter and are summarized in Table 4.17 and Figure 4.18. The home planned group is now split into columns 1 and 3 on this table. The epidural and spinal analgesia rates were highest among the transfers who had to go to hospital while the pethidine users were less represented in the transferred group. The proportions of non-pharmacological method users were about the same among those who remained at home and those who were transferred. This was probably because the latter group of women had already used these methods before the need of transfer to hospital became apparent.

Regional analysis of pain relief produced many boxes with small numbers in some areas, e.g. aromatherapy, homeopathy and acupuncture. Outstanding were the wider ranges of all pharmacological analgesics in home and hospital, nitrous oxide and pethidine 9–65% in the home and 53–83% in the hospital. Less than 10% had no analgesia in the hospital booked/hospital delivered group with the exception of Oxford when 13% had none. Conversely the average of 17% with no analgesia in home births included some very high rates in Scotland (31%) and West Midlands (22%).

Table 4.17 The analgesic methods used by 3922 women planning and delivering at home, 3319 planning to have a hospital delivery and 769 who had to transfer to hospital from home reported by midwives. More than one method was used often so totals >100%. (NBTF Home Births Survey 1994)

	Planned and delivered at home		Planned and delivered in hospital		Planned home birth but delivered in hospital	
	n	%	*n*	%	*n*	%
Pharmacological methods						
Nitrous oxide	1948	50.1	2405	72.7	499	65.8
Pethidine	169	4.3	1013	30.6	180	23.7
Epidural	1**	—	377	11.4	136	17.9
Spinal	2**	—	42	1.3	31	4.1
Non-pharmacological methods						
Relaxation	1953	50.3	988	29.9	327	43.1
TENS*	801	20.6	511	15.5	218	28.8
Warm water	951	24.5	266	8.0	182	24.0
Aromatherapy	203	5.2	19	0.9	39	5.1
Homeopathy	128	3.3	9	0.3	30	4.0
Acupuncture	21	0.5	1	—	7	0.9
None	731	18.8	273	8.3	60	7.9
Not known/ reported	10		13		11	

*TENS, transcutaneous electrical nerve stimulation
**Not used for labour

COMPLICATIONS IN LABOUR

Among the women who had booked at home and stayed there for delivery, a small number had labour complications. This was an open ended question so we learn only of those things the midwife wished to report. For example, 40 women of the 3896 who delivered at home were reported here with a prolonged labour and 130 had fetal distress.

Among all the women who planned to deliver at home there were 221 and 254 with these complications respectively. Hence of those with prolonged labour about 181 (82%) were moved for a hospital delivery and among those with fetal distress about a half similarly were transported before delivery. Shoulder dystocia was reported in 45 of those who planned to deliver at home and 34 of those who actually did; the closeness of these two numbers is understandable for shoulder dystocia is a complication that allows no time to get help from a hospital unit and

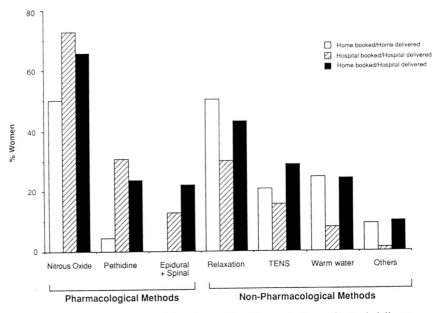

Figure 4.18 The analgesia used by place of booking and place of actual delivery. More than one method was sometimes used by one woman (NBTF Home Births Survey 1994)

treatment must be given on the spot by those who are available. These were the major problems reported and they occurred in 6% of all the home planned/home delivered women.

By comparison in the hospital group, 18% had a complication in labour. Table 4.18 shows that whilst shoulder dystocia rates are about the same, that of prolonged labour was reported four times more often and fetal distress three times increased.

The group who were home planned/hospital delivered had a very much higher rate of complications with 41% of them reporting problems. Again shoulder dystocia is not greatly increased because it had to be dealt with in the home but prolonged labour was 25 times increased and fetal distress was four times higher. One could not judge from the answers that this was the only reason for the admission to hospital.

Prolapsed cord was not reported once in the home planned/home delivered group (3896) nor in the hospital planned/hospital delivered women (3319). One should not be surprised at this low rate of prolapse of the cord. While presentation of the cord may be in found in 1:300 women in labour and prolapse may follow in about a third of these (i.e. 1:900), the women in this study would under-represent the higher risk groups for

Table 4.18 Complications in labour reported by midwives (NBTF Home Births Survey 1994)

	Planned and delivered at home (n = 3922)		Planned and delivered in hospital (n = 3319)		Planned home birth but delivered in hospital (n = 769)	
	n	%	n	%	n	%
Fetal distress	130	3.4	351	10.8	124	16.2
Prolonged labour	40	0.9	130	4.0	181	23.3
Shoulder dystocia	34	0.8	31	1.0	11	1.4
Not known/recorded	32		45		26	

cord prolapse – breech and transverse presentations, very small babies and those with polyhydramnios. One woman only in the home booked/hospital delivered group had a prolapsed cord but no fetal death was reported. It is probable that with those conditions where time for transfer allowed, women were moved in for hospital care.

WOMEN TRANSFERRED TO HOSPITAL AFTER A HOME BOOKING

Whilst this group has been referred to previously in many places in this chapter, we performed a separate fuller analysis, for these women always raise questions.

The reasons for transfer to hospital care are summarized in Table 4.19. The reasons exceed the numbers of women for more than one indication for transfer was often recorded.

The majority of women (79%) were transferred for reasons related to labour and delivery. Table 4.20 analyses the interval between transfer and delivery. The most important factor determining a woman not delivering at home after having been booked for a home birth was parity. Nulliparity was associated with a highly significant increase in the risk of hospital birth. Only 60% of nulliparae achieved their desire for a home birth compared with 90% of multiparae. Previous delivery by Caesarean section was also a risk factor for transfer to hospital care; 4% of multiparae were transferred to hospital care having a previous Caesarean section compared with 1% of those who delivered at home as intended.

The main reported reasons for transfer to hospital were problems related to labour of which prolonged labour was the commonest in 39% of

Table 4.19 Reasons given for transfer to hospital reported by women (NBTF Home Births Survey 1994); more than one reason was given ($n = 896$)

Reason given	n	%
High blood pressure	69	7.7
Haemorrhage	65	7.3
Intrauterine growth retardation	19	2.1
Fetal distress	131	14.6
No progress	333	37.2
Premature rupture of membranes	222	24.8
Cord prolapse	1	0.1
Assessment	54	6.0
Intrauterine death	2	0.2

Table 4.20 Comparison of timing and reason for transfer reported by midwives (NBTF Home Births Survey 1994)

Reason for transfer	Before labour	During labour	After the birth
Prolonged labour	0	189	0
Malpresentation	0	24	0
Antepartum haemorrhage	1	5	0
Postpartum haemorrhage	0	0	28
Retained placenta	0	0	22
Bad 2nd/3rd degree tear	0	0	7
Dystocia	0	8	0
Hypertension	9	10	0
Abdominal pain	2	0	0
Premature rupture of membranes	15	7	0
Total	27	243	57

cases. Table 4.2 summarizes the total duration of the first stage of labour by place of birth in all women.

Twenty-nine per cent of all women who required transfer to hospital had a first stage of labour lasting more than 12 h compared with only less than 7% of those delivering at home or in hospital as intended. Sixty-three per cent of these were primigravidae. The first stage lasted more than 12 h in 48% of primigravidae who were transferred from home to hospital care compared with 17% of those who delivered in hospital as planned and 21% of those who delivered at home as planned.

Delay in the second stage of labour was also more common in this group (see Table 4.3) with 20% of women who required transfer from home to hospital having a second stage of more than 2 h, compared with only 5% of those who delivered in hospital as planned and only 2% of those who delivered at home as planned. Eighty-six per cent of these women who experienced a second stage of more than 2 h and were transferred from home to hospital were primigravidae.

MANAGEMENT

The treatment received in hospital following transfer was consistent with the indications for transfer (Table 4.21).

Analysis of the method of delivery by intended place of birth shows that intended hospital delivery is associated with a twofold increase in the likelihood of both assisted vaginal delivery and Caesarean section (Table 4.22).

No assisted vaginal deliveries or, obviously, Caesarean sections were performed at home, so these interventions were concentrated in the group who were transferred to hospital. The instrumental vaginal delivery rate was 17% in this group overall and 30% in primigravidae. The Caesarean section rate was 15% in the transferred group overall and 16% in primigravidae.

Given the high incidence of prolonged labour and acceleration of labour in the women transferred to hospital, it is not surprising that some of these women needed epidural analgesia. The overall rate of epidural analgesia in this group was 12% with a 30% rate in primigravidae. These rates were almost identical to those in women who delivered in hospital as planned (12% overall and 33% in the primigravidae).

TRANSFER TO HOSPITAL

Midwives caring for women who were transferred to hospital recorded the interval between requesting help and its actual arrival (Table 4.23). Help arrived within 15 min in 50% of cases and within 1 h in 98% of cases.

Professional support was provided during transfer. The midwife caring for the woman at home accompanied her to hospital in 61% of cases. The method of transport is summarized in Table 4.24.

The journey to hospital took less than 30 min in the majority of cases (Table 4.25).

It appears that when the midwife accompanied the woman to hospital, she stayed on to attend the delivery in many cases. Fifty-five per cent of the women who were transferred to hospital reported that a familiar

Table 4.21 Treatment received in hospital following transfer reported by women (NBTF Home Births Survey 1994)

Treatment	n	%
Drip to accelerate labour	292	32.7
Induction of labour	206	23.1
Forceps/vacuum	121	13.6
Caesarean section	100	11.2
Blood transfusion	22	2.5
Removal of placenta	104	11.7
Repair of tear	260	29.1
None	165	18.5

Table 4.22 Mode of delivery by intended place of birth reported by midwives (NBTF Home Births Survey 1994)

Mode of delivery	Planned home birth		Planned hospital birth	
	n	%	n	%
Spontaneous cephalic	4414	94.5	3001	89.7
Other spontaneous	30	0.6	17	0.5
Assisted vaginal	115	2.5	180	5.5
Caesarean section	94	2.0	139	4.2

midwife was present at the birth compared with 84% of those who delivered at home as planned and 32% of those delivering in hospital as planned. In 97% of cases women were pleased by the presence of the familiar midwife:

> Admission to hospital was much less traumatic as our midwife came with us and delivered the baby.

SATISFACTION

When questioned immediately after the event, transfer to hospital was an upsetting event for 59% of women, while 41% did not find it at all upsetting.

However, despite this distress, the majority of women (89%) accepted the reasons given for transfer to hospital:

Table 4.23 Arrival of help reported by midwives (NBTF Home Births Survey 1994)

Time	n	%
<5 min	25	6.8
5–15 min	158	43.1
16–60 min	175	47.7
1–2 h	6	1.6
2–4 h	2	0.5
>4 h	1	0.3

Table 4.24 Method of transfer reported by midwives (NBTF Home Births Survey 1994)

Method of transfer	n	%
Obstetric flying squad	3	0.4
Neonatal flying squad	1	0.1
Ambulance with paramedics	99	12.9
Ambulance with midwife	139	18.1
Ambulance with midwife and paramedics	137	17.9
Car	377	49.2
Helicopter/plane	1	0.1
Ambulance only	8	1.0
Ambulance with GP	2	0.3

Table 4.25 Duration of journey to hospital reported by midwives (NBTF Home Births Survey 1994)

Time	n	%
<10 min	101	18.2
10–30 min	416	74.8
31–59 min	33	5.9
1–5 h	6	1.1

> I did not regret planning a home birth and felt confident in the midwives' decision to transfer me to hospital and in the decision to have a Caesarean section.

> I wished to have a home birth, but due to circumstances beyond my control that could not happen. The thing I appreciated most was that this was not seen as a failure on anyone's account.

However, 5% disagreed, feeling transfer was due to anxiety on the part of the midwife or doctor:

> I felt the inducement [sic] was partially manufactured to prevent me staying at home.

> My GP was happy to do home delivery until it actually happened, then he panicked terribly ... scared a lot of people unnecessarily.

Inevitably, the eventual level of satisfaction was influenced by the outcome. In all groups of women the level of satisfaction with midwifery care was very high. However, women who were transferred from home to hospital were more likely to be dissatisfied with their care.

> Hospital midwives not caring like community, you feel like a piece of meat.

These women were more likely to come into contact with doctors at the time of birth than either of the other two groups and expressed less satisfaction with the care received from them. This is shown in detail in Chapter 9.

Another method of judging satisfaction is the expressed preference for place of birth in any further pregnancies. As reported in Chapter 9, a very high percentage of all groups hoped to deliver in the same place as they had planned in the index pregnancy. In the home planned/home delivered group 98% wished to have their next baby at home. Some 93% of the hospital booked/hospital delivered group wished to go to hospital for their next baby, but women who were transferred from home to hospital (11%) were much more likely to consider a change of plan for the next pregnancy from planning a home birth to a hospital booked one. Among those who wished to have the next baby in hospital, almost half had been transferred because of prolonged labour.

CONCLUSION

Complex data are reported here and need careful interpretation. Often more than one factor exists and emphasis may have resulted from the questions asked on the preformed questionnaire. Generally booked home births had a straightforward, well-covered delivery with appropriate care. Those transferred to hospital in labour deserve careful scrutiny to see if any tightening of the acceptance criteria for a home birth could have reduced this 16% of increased anxiety. The position of primigravida obviously needs more examination since 40% had to be transferred from the home delivery they had hoped and planned for.

REFERENCES

1. Prendiville, W.J. and Elbourne, D.R. (1995). Prophylactic oxytocics in third stage of labour. [revised 1 April 1993]. In Keirse, M.J., Renfrew, M.J., Neilson, J.P. and Crowther, C. (eds.) *Pregnancy and Childbirth Database* [database on disk and CDROM]. The Cochrane Collaboration; Issue 2, Oxford: Update Software; 1995. Available from BMJ Publishing Group, London
2. Begley, C.M. (1990). A comparison of active and physiological management of the third stage of labour. *Midwifery,* **6**, 3–17
3. Prendiville, W.J., Harding, J.E., Elbourne, D.R. and Stirrat, G.M. (1988). The Bristol third stage trial: active vs. physiological management of third stage of labour. *Br. Med. J.,* **297**, 1295–1300
4. Chamberlain, G. and Gunn, P. (1987). *Birthplace.* (Chichester: John Wiley)
5. Hodnett, E.D. (1996). Support from caregivers during childbirth. In Enkin, M.W., Keirse, M.J., Renfrew, M.J. and Neilson, J.P. (eds.) *Pregnancy and Childbirth Module of the Cochrane Database of Systematic Reviews, 1996* [updated 29 February 1996]. Available in the Cochrane Library from BMJ Publishing Group, London
6. Anderson, G.M. and Lomas, J. (1985). Determinants of the increasing Caesarean birth rate: Ontario Data 1979–1982. *N. Engl. J. Med.,* **311**, 887–92

5

After the delivery

PROBLEMS REPORTED BY THE MOTHER

The data in this section come mostly from the questionnaires which the mothers themselves completed. Hence some totals are slightly different from the previous section where midwives' questionnaires were largely used. Many symptoms are subjective and hence the critical level of reporting differs from one woman to another. Allowing for the differences of populations giving birth in hospital and the home, they may be used in a general way to give some indication of the woman's state in the first 48 h after delivery.

The complaints for the women who were home booked/home delivered were fewer than those in the hospital group and considerably less than those who, having booked for home, had to transfer to hospital. This is understandable for amongst the last group were the highest incidence of complications and interventions; there must be many disappointed women who had hoped to deliver at home and disappointment often makes symptoms worse.

Examining one of the symptoms: tiredness shows a gradient from the home group at 67%, the hospital of 77% and those delivered in hospital having booked at home to 78%. This is not surprising for hospital does not provide the best environment for rest. It is a noisy communal place. Tearfulness, piles and constipation follow the same trend but backache was very much greater in the hospital booked/hospital delivered group at 43% compared with 34% in the other groups. Headaches conversely have a lower representation in the home booked/home delivered group with only 8% compared with 11% in the other groups. Breast problems were

Table 5.1 Problems reported by the mother in the first 48 h after delivery. Some women reported several problems and as the percentages are of the women reporting each problem, they would add to more than 100% (NBTF Home Births Survey 1994)

	Planned and delivered at home (n = 4191)		Planned and delivered in hospital (n = 3470)		Planned home but deliverd in hospital (n = 809)	
	n	%	n	%	n	%
Tiredness	2817	67.6	2671	77.4	629	78.4
Tearfulness	517	12.4	632	18.3	203	25.3
Backache	1425	32.2	1495	43.3	278	34.7
Headache	311	7.5	385	11.2	84	10.5
Piles	584	14.0	591	17.1	170	21.9
Constipation	476	11.4	434	12.6	132	16.5
Painful sutures	339	8.1	838	24.3	208	25.9
Afterpains in uterus	293	7.0	211	6.1	27	3.4
Breast problems	488	11.7	394	11.4	115	14.3
Other problems	351	8.4	525	15.1	163	20.2
Not known/ reported	26		14		4	

about the same in all groups as were uterine afterpains but painful sutures were reported considerably less frequently in the home booked/home delivered group at 8% compared with the hospital group which was three times as great both among those booked and those unbooked for delivery in hospital; only 52% of the home delivered had perineal damage compared with 62% in the hospital group.

It is difficult to draw too many conclusions from Table 5.1 but it would seem that those who had been booked for and delivered at home were a more satisfied group of women.

BLOOD LOSS AND THE MANUAL REMOVAL OF PLACENTA

Among the home group, blood loss of less then 200 ml was reported in 75% compared with 65% of hospital booked/hospital delivered and 53% of home booked/hospital delivered groups. Similarly, reports of blood loss above 500 ml, the definition of primary postpartum haemorrhage, was 4% (hospital booked/hospital delivered, 2% (home booked/home delivered) and 9% (home booked/hospital delivered) a five times greater proportion among those transferred.

There is a trend towards a correlation between blood loss and the management of the third stage.

Table 5.2 Blood loss by method of placental delivery (NBTF Home Births Survey 1994)

	Home planned/home delivered						Hospital planned/hospital delivered					
	Physiological (n = 1595)		Controlled cord traction (n = 2165)		Manual removal (n = 28)		Physiological (n = 178)		Controlled cord traction (n = 2757)		Manual removal (n = 90)	
Blood loss (ml)	n	%	n	%	n	%	n	%	n	%	n	%
≤200	1090	69	1664	77	11	39	114	64	1739	67	13	15
201–500	467	29	473	22	11	39	51	29	820	30	46	51
> 500*	38	2	28	1	6	21	13	7	98	4	31	34

*>500 ml is the definition of primary postpartum haemorrhage

Table 5.2 shows that the postpartum haemorrhage rate was low for both non-interventional methods and controlled cord traction although both methods were associated with a higher rate in hospital 7% and 4% compared with 2% and 1% in the home. The higher rates of 21% and 34% associated with manual removal might have been due to the indication for the procedure.

Responses about those who had their placentae delivered by non-interventional physiological methods were reanalysed for a number had been given an oxytocic. We do not know when their oxytocic was given, but since the placental delivery was described as physiological, we considered it was given later and not prophylactically. Even those with the least loss (less than 200 ml) had syntometrine, syntocinon, or oxytocin in 5% and 12% respectively of home and hospital deliveries. These proportions were 29% and 38% in association with a postpartum haemorrhage. It is noticeable that 27 of 38 women who had a postpartum haemorrhage at home were not reported as receiving any oxytocic; a similar deficit occurred in eight out of 13 hospital births with physiological placental deliveries.

A similar gradient is found on those who had a manual removal of the placenta. Respectively 30 (1%), 97 (3%) and 51 (7%) had this procedure, an eightfold increase in the hospital delivered over the home delivered/ home booking group.

PERINEAL PROBLEMS

The data reported in the study about perineal damage and repair have been analysed and are reported in Tables 5.4 to 5.10. There is a discrepancy in

Table 5.3 Blood loss among those who had a physiological delivery by the use of an oxytocic drug (syntometrine, syntocinon or oxytocin) (NBTF Home Births Survey 1994)

	Home planned/home delivered			Hospital planned/hospital delivered		
	No oxytocic (*n* = 1478)	*With oxytocic* (*n* = 107)	*% of total receiving*	*No oxytocic* (*n* = 150)	*With oxytocic* (*n* = 28)	*% of total receiving*
Blood loss (ml)	*n* *%*	*n* *%*	*oxytocic*	*n* *%*	*n* *%*	*oxytocic*
≤200	1035 70	55 51	5	100 67	14 50	12
201–500	416 28	41 38	9	42 28	9 32	18
>500*	27 2	11 10	29	8 5	5 18	38

*>500 ml is definition of postpartum haemorrhage

the totals between the details of the repair and the numbers of those reporting any damage. This is probably because a large number of first-degree tears and small vaginal wall repairs did not need suturing, a common finding with many deliveries.

Perineal damage is reported in Table 5.4. Of those who delivered at home, 48% reported having no damage compared with 39% of the hospital group. The transferred group had an intermediate figure at 42%. While to some extent this might be due to the easier births in the home delivery group, it could also imply careful deliveries by the midwives. The midwives at the home deliveries were more senior and therefore probably more experienced than many of the hospital midwives. Over twice the number of G grade midwives were the lead professionals at home compared with hospital.

Among those in whom perineal damage was reported, the degree of trauma varied so there was a greater proportion of first-degree tears in the home delivery group than in the others but the second-degree tears were about the same ratio. The third-degree tears occurred rarely in each group being highest in those delivered in hospital. There were only four cervical tears reported in the survey and they all occurred in hospital deliveries.

A significant difference ($p < 0.0001$) occurred in the episiotomies. In the home group only 4% of women had episiotomy while 21% in the hospital planned/hospital delivered group and 34% in the home planned/hospital delivered group had episiotomies. This would equate with the vaginal operative deliveries and increased length of second stage of labour in these groups.

It was mostly midwives who repaired the perineum at each site. Figure 5.1 shows the regional difference; excluding the Celtic kingdoms the

Table 5.4 Perineal damage reported by midwives (NBTF Home Births Study 1994). Multiple answers were allowed. This is reported incidents not women and so no totals are provided.

	Planned and delivered at home		Planned and delivered in hospital		Planned home but deliverd in hospital	
	n	%	*n*	%	*n*	%
First-degree tear	918	45.2	650	31.4	94	21.3
Second-degree tear	798	39.3	783	39.8	149	33.9
Third-degree tear	4	0.2	13	0.6	3	0.7
Vaginal wall only	222	10.9	184	8.9	46	10.4
Cervical tear	0	0	3	0.1	1	0.2
Episiotomy	89	4.3	435	21.0	149	33.9
Not known/recorded	15		20		22	
Subtotal with damage	2031	52	2068	61	442	58
Subtotal without damage	1882	48	1293	39	316	42

lower proportions of midwife suturing are associated with higher general practitioner activity in home births. At home, the midwives who repaired were those who actually did the delivery in over half of instances (Table 5.5). In the home group 76% of repairs were performed by midwives, a similar proportion to the hospital group – 71%. Of those transferred from home to hospital 51% were repaired by midwives; 48% were repaired by doctors, twice the proportion of doctor repairs compared with the other two groups. This probably reflects again the increased proportion of operative deliveries by doctors that took place in the higher risk group who were transferred from home.

The personnel who repaired the perineum in the regions is reported in Tables 5.6, 5.7 and 5.8 which refer respectively to women who were home booked/home delivered, hospital booked/hospital delivered, and home booked/hospital delivered. In Table 5.6 the delivering midwife did the repair in only four regions more than 70% of the time while in six regions this happened less than half the time. Since a second midwife was usually present it is not surprising that the load was shared between the midwives to some extent. The general practitioner, having not been the lead professional at delivery in many deliveries (see Chapter 4) was involved in perineal repairs up to 40% of the time in two regions. This shows the wide range of load that is generated in domiciliary deliveries.

There was some reporting of women who, having given birth at home, were transferred into hospital for repair of perineum. The reason given

Table 5.5 Who repaired the perineum reported by midwives (NBTF Home Births Survey 1994)

Repair by:	Planned and delivered at home		Planned and delivered in hospital		Planned home but delivered in hospital	
	n	%	n	%	n	%
Midwife						
who delivered	564	57.3	779	49.2	118	33.7
another	181	18.4	350	22.1	62	17.7
Subtotal	745	75.7	1129	71.3	180	51.4
Doctor*						
GP	206	20.9	40	2.5	10	2.8
SHO	12	1.2	182	11.5	43	12.3
registrar	22	2.2	216	13.7	112	32.0
consultant	0	—	14	0.9	5	1.4
Subtotal	240	24.3	452	27.6	170	48.6
Not known/reported	16		20		23	
Total	985		1581		350	

*GP, general practitioner; SHO, senior house officer

Table 5.6 Personnel who repaired the perineum by region, planned home/delivered home reported by midwives (NBTF Home Births Survey 1994)

Region	Midwife who delivered		Other midwife		General practitioner		Other doctor	
	n	%	n	%	n	%	n	%
Northern	8	40.0	3	15.0	5	25.0	4	20.0
Yorkshire	26	50.9	4	7.8	20	39.2	1	1.9
Trent	23	42.5	13	24.0	14	25.9	4	7.4
East Anglia	34	46.5	7	9.6	30	41.0	2	2.6
North West Thames	36	65.4	10	18.1	7	12.7	2	3.6
North East Thames	42	72.4	9	15.5	3	5.1	4	6.8
South East Thames	48	54.5	24	27.2	14	15.9	2	2.2
South West Thames	39	63.9	16	26.2	5	8.2	1	1.6
Wessex	35	66.0	6	11.3	8	15.0	4	7.5
Oxford	35	51.5	10	14.7	22	32.3	1	1.5
South Western	33	43.4	17	22.4	25	32.9	1	1.3
West Midlands	49	70.0	17	24.3	4	5.7	0	—
Mersey	13	72.2	1	5.6	4	22.2	0	—
North Western	35	71.4	4	8.2	8	16.3	1	2.0
Northern Ireland	1	12.5	0	—	7	87.5	0	—
Scotland	14	32.5	10	23.2	14	32.5	4	9.3
Wales	37	68.5	11	20.4	5	9.2	1	1.9
Total	508	56.6	162	18.0	195	21.7	32	3.7

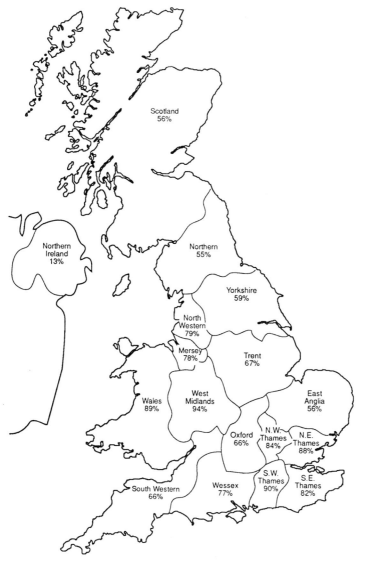

Figure 5.1 Percentage of perineal repairs done by midwives; home planned/home delivered women (NBTF Home Births Survey 1994)

Table 5.7 Personnel who repaired the perineum by region, planned hospital/delivered hospital reported by midwives (NBTF Home Births Survey 1994)

Region	Midwife who delivered		Other midwife		Senior house officer		Registrar		Consultant	
	n	%	*n*	%	*n*	%	*n*	%	*n*	%
Northern	26	5.9	4	9.0	7	15.9	5	11.4	0	—
Yorkshire	44	62.0	9	12.6	14	19.7	3	4.2	0	—
Trent	30	40.5	19	25.6	13	17.5	8	10.8	0	—
East Anglia	58	63.7	18	19.8	2	2.2	11	12.0	0	—
North West Thames	41	46.5	17	19.3	18	20.4	12	13.6	0	—
North East Thames	33	54.0	10	16.4	8	13.1	9	14.7	1	1.6
South East Thames	41	39.8	33	32.0	15	14.3	13	12.6	1	0.9
South West Thames	28	48.2	16	27.5	6	10.3	7	12.0	0	—
Wessex	32	51.6	17	27.4	6	9.6	6	9.6	0	—
Oxford	43	43.4	27	27.2	9	9.0	10	10.1	2	2.0
South Western	52	41.2	37	29.3	10	7.9	22	17.4	0	—
West Midlands	66	61.1	21	19.4	7	6.5	13	12.0	0	—
Mersey	16	61.5	2	7.7	3	11.5	5	19.2	0	—
North Western	45	56.2	12	15.0	8	10.0	11	13.7	1	1.2
Northern Ireland	6	42.8	3	21.4	2	14.3	0	—	2	14.3
Scotland	45	47.8	19	20.2	5	5.3	16	17.0	2	2.1
Wales	54	63.5	13	15.3	6	7.0	9	10.5	1	1.1
Total	660	53.0	277	22.2	139	11.2	160	12.8	10	0.8

was not always the extent of the damage but the lack of expertise, as one midwife commented :

> The mother was transferred to hospital for repair of laceration – reason being midwives on duty were not up to date on suturing. GP informed but he also was not up to date. Hospital was asked for assistance – unable to provide this therefore mother had to be transferred.

In hospital booked/hospital delivered women (Table 5.7) midwives still did the majority of repairs, 53% being the delivery midwife and 22% another. There is an inverse ratio between midwives and the hospital doctors which shows interesting variations in the regions. For example, in East Anglia midwives repaired 84% and doctors 14% while in North East Thames, 70% of midwives and 29% of doctors did the suturing. Other regions fell between these two ends of the range.

Women booked for home but transferred to hospital showed a greater proportion of repairs by registrars and senior registrars but the numbers in each box are small and so the figures in Table 5.8 are given for completeness and no statistical trends have been sought.

Table 5.8 Personnel who repaired the perineum by region, planned home/delivered hospital reported by midwives (NBTF Home Births Survey 1994)

Region	Midwife who delivered		Other midwife		Senior house officer		Registrar		Consultant	
	n	%	n	%	n	%	n	%	n	%
Northern	8	66.6	2	16.7	1	8.4	1	8.4	0	—
Yorkshire	10	45.5	3	13.6	3	13.6	4	18.2	0	—
Trent	2	15.4	1	7.7	3	23.0	6	46.1	0	—
East Anglia	5	27.8	4	22.2	1	5.5	7	38.9	0	—
North West Thames	3	25.0	2	16.7	0	—	6	50.0	0	—
North East Thames	3	16.7	1	5.6	4	22.2	10	55.6	0	—
South East Thames	9	33.3	6	22.2	4	14.8	8	29.6	0	—
South West Thames	7	36.8	6	31.5	2	10.5	2	10.5	0	—
Wessex	9	50.0	1	5.5	1	5.5	6	33.5	0	—
Oxford	4	33.4	1	8.2	3	25.0	4	33.4	0	—
South Western	8	28.6	4	14.3	3	10.7	13	46.4	0	—
West Midlands	9	36.0	5	20.0	1	4.0	8	32.0	2	8.0
Mersey	2	40.0	1	20.0	1	20.0	0	—	0	—
North Western	2	22.3	4	44.5	1	11.1	2	22.3	0	—
Northern Ireland	0	—	0	—	0	—	0	—	0	—
Scotland	5	21.7	6	26.0	0	—	8	34.8	1	4.3
Wales	5	33.3	1	6.6	5	33.3	4	26.6	0	—
Total	91	34.5	48	18.2	33	12.5	89	33.8	3	0.2

Table 5.9 and Figure 5.2 give the time taken from delivery to repair, a matter of concern felt by many women who dread having to wait a long time for their sutures. This was derived from the questions which asked the actual time of delivery and the time at which the repair took place. Most repairs were promptly done, half were within 15 minutes and 70% within half an hour. Amongst the group transferred from home to hospital there was a trend towards more delay, possibly because of the transfer.

The material used for repair was slightly better reported than the information on those who did the repairs and is shown in Table 5.10 and Figure 5.3. In the home group 63% were repaired with catgut and another 28% were with man-made absorbable materials. This is disappointing in view of the known superiority of polyglycol stitches over catgut, with its concomitant lower complication rate[1].

A different picture is seen in the hospital group where 54% were sutured with catgut and 40% had polyglycol sutures. An even higher proportion of the new man-made suturing materials were used amongst those who were transferred from home to hospital, an overall report of 46% women. This might be associated with the fact that more senior

Table 5.9 The time interval from delivery to repair of perineum reported by midwives (NBTF Home Births Survey 1994)

Time taken	Planned and delivered at home		Planned and delivered in hospital		Planned home but delivered in hospital	
	n	%	n	%	n	%
<15 min	434	46.1	704	46.8	174	52.9
15–30 min	229	24.3	309	20.6	61	18.5
31–60 min	185	19.7	300	20.0	60	18.2
61–180 min (1–3 h)	81	8.6	181	12.0	20	6.1
181–720 min (3–6 h)	10	1.1	3	0.2	1	0.3
>720 min (>6 h)	2	0.2	6	0.4	4	1.2
Not known/recorded	2955		1530		320	
Total	941		1503		330	

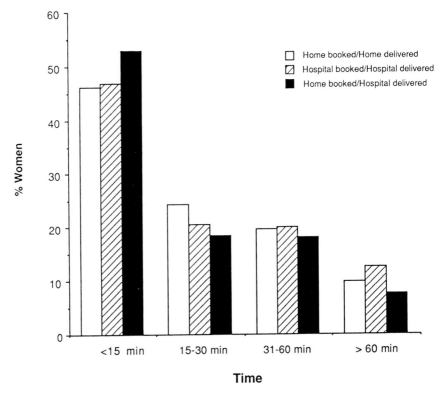

Figure 5.2 The time interval from delivery to repair of perineum (NBTF Home Births Survey 1994)

Table 5.10 The materials used for perineal suture reported by midwives (NBTF Home Births Survey 1994)

	Planned and delivered at home		Planned and delivered in hospital		Planned home but delivered in hospital	
	n	%	n	%	n	%
Catgut	658	63.4	914	54.4	178	49.2
Silk	69	6.6	61	3.6	10	2.8
Dexon/Vicryl	288	27.8	672	39.9	165	45.9
Other	23	0.2	32	1.9	9	2.5
Not known/recorded	22		25		25	
Total	1038		1679		362	

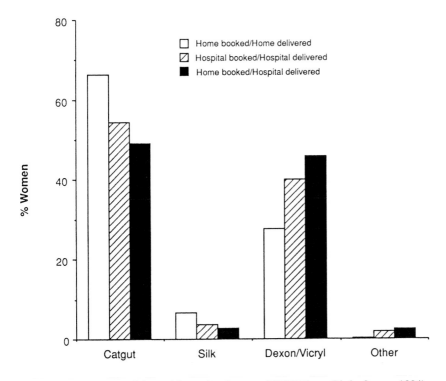

Figure 5.3 The materials used for perineal suture (NBTF Home Births Survey 1994)

Table 5.11 Use of suture material by regions – home booked/home delivered reported by midwives (NBTF Home Births Survey 1994)

Region	Catgut		Dexon & Vicryl		Silk		Other	
	n	%	*n*	%	*n*	%	*n*	%
Northern	17	62.9	6	22.2	4	14.8	0	—
Yorkshire	35	62.5	15	26.8	6	10.7	0	—
Trent	28	49.1	24	42.0	4	7.0	1	1.8
East Anglia	49	68.0	22	30.4	1	1.4	0	—
North West Thames	33	58.9	22	39.3	0	—	1	1.8
North East Thames	41	70.7	17	29.3	0	—	0	—
South East Thames	59	67.0	25	28.4	0	—	4	4.6
South West Thames	48	77.4	13	21.0	1	1.6	0	—
Wessex	48	84.2	2	3.5	6	10.5	1	1.8
Oxford	56	76.7	7	9.5	7	9.6	3	4.1
South Western	45	52.9	24	28.2	11	12.9	5	5.9
West Midlands	52	66.7	15	19.2	10	12.8	1	1.3
Mersey	15	83.3	3	16.7	0	—	0	—
North Western	16	31.4	32	62.6	2	3.9	1	2.0
Northern Ireland	6	50.0	1	8.4	5	4.6	0	—
Scotland	13	30.2	26	60.4	4	9.3	0	—
Wales	42	71.2	11	18.6	3	5.0	3	5.0

Table 5.12 Use of suture materials by regions – hospital booked/hospital delivered (NBTF Home Births Survey 1994)

Region	Catgut		Dexon & Vicryl		Silk		Other	
	n	%	*n*	%	*n*	%	*n*	%
Northern	25	45.5	21	38.1	9	16.4	0	—
Yorkshire	29	36.7	43	54.3	4	5.0	3	3.8
Trent	30	37.5	48	59.9	1	1.2	1	1.2
East Anglia	52	57.1	39	42.7	0	—	0	—
North West Thames	43	47.8	47	52.2	0	—	0	—
North East Thames	32	50.8	30	47.6	1	1.6	0	—
South East Thames	63	60.0	39	37.1	1	0.9	2	1.9
South West Thames	47	81.0	11	19.0	0	—	0	—
Wessex	57	91.9	2	3.2	0	—	3	4.8
Oxford	69	62.7	28	33.5	13	11.8	0	—
South Western	75	55.1	55	14.7	2	1.4	4	2.9
West Midlands	84	72.4	20	17.2	9	7.7	3	2.6
Mersey	20	80.0	5	20.0	0	—	0	—
North Western	30	34.9	49	57.0	1	1.2	6	6.9
Northern Ireland	5	26.3	9	47.3	5	26.3	0	—
Scotland	19	20.2	74	78.6	1	1.0	1	1.0
Wales	50	56.8	36	40.6	1	1.1	1	1.1

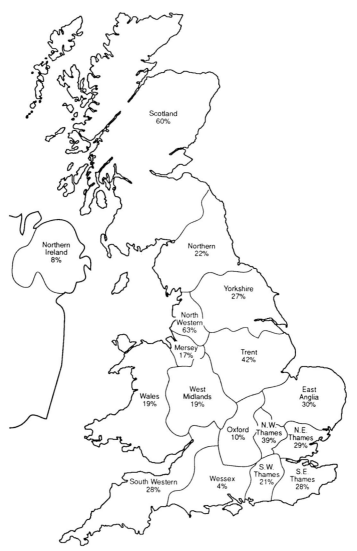

Figure 5.4 Percentage of use by repair of Dexon/Vicryl by regions; home booked/home delivered (NBTF Home Births Survey 1994)

doctors were involved with repair of these perineums and these might have been more aware of the advantages of polyglycol.

Another sad finding is that silk is still being used in a significant proportion of perineum repairs – 7% in the home, 4% in the hospital and 3% in the home transferred to hospital. These sutures are uncomfortable and have to be removed later. One had hoped that inabsorbable sutures had mostly gone from UK use by 1994. A very small number might have been because of an extensive irregular tear which the operator felt would heal better with fine silk stitches carefully placed in the skin but there is little place for inabsorbable stitches in the perineum after delivery. In the home birth group, 36 of the 69 repairs done with silk were performed by the general practitioner.

Breakdown of these data by region shows some to be using catgut in over 75% of cases at home (Wessex, South West Thames, Mersey and Oxford) while man-made absorbables had a converse proportion (Table 5.11 and Figure 5.4). Silk at home deliveries was used in more than 10% in five regions – Wessex, South Western, Northern, Yorkshire and West Midlands regions. The proportions for those delivering in hospital are not uniform in the regions (Table 5.12). Five are reporting a use of man-made absorbable sutures in over 50% of cases – North West Thames, Yorkshire, Trent, North Western and Scotland but although numbers are small, three regions still suture with silk in the hospital, Northern, Oxford and Northern Ireland in more than 10% of women.

CONCLUSIONS

Generally the home delivered group has fewer problems than the hospital group. The trends of placental delivery indicate a lower use of oxytocics on home deliveries. This applies both to the prophylactic use to prevent a postpartum haemorrhage and in the treatment of heavy blood loss. Episiotomies were fewer but first-degree tears were increased in the home. Repair was mostly in the hands of midwives and was promptly performed. There is still a large use of catgut rather than man-made absorbable sutures; this is both at home and in hospital.

REFERENCE

1. Mahomed, K., Grant, A.M., Ashurst, H. and James, D. (1989). The Southmead perineal suture study. A randomised comparison of suture materials and suturing techniques for repair of perineal trauma. *Br. J. Obstet. Gynaecol.*, **96**, 1272–80

6

The baby

OUTCOME

Perinatal mortality

The outcome for the baby is often measured in comparative perinatal mortality rates (PNMR). These data include the stillbirths occurring after the 24th completed week of pregnancy and the first-week neonatal deaths. It is an inexact guide, in Western countries often owing more to biological and genetic background than to measuring the services and facilities provided in pregnancy or labour. In this study so few perinatal deaths were reported that the comparison between the groups is insubstantial. There was one neonatal death and no stillbirths in the home booked/ home delivered group (3896 women), four stillbirths and one death in the hospital booked/hospital delivered group (3319 women) and two stillbirths and two neonatal deaths in the home booked/hospital delivered group (769 women). There were also three deaths (one stillbirth and two neonatal deaths) in the smaller group of women who had registered in the study but did not return their questionnaires (379 women). These figures are very small compared with the national perinatal mortality rate of about eight per thousand total births.

One must reiterate that this survey was basically about women who had booked by 37 weeks of pregnancy for a home delivery. Hence they joined the study before outcome was known and so avoided bias but by setting 37 weeks of gestation as a dividing line, most who were going to have preterm births with their greater perinatal risks were excluded from the study. We know of only 53 women of 3896 in the planned home group who delivered before 37 weeks. Hence those left after 37 weeks must be at a lower risk than the total population owing to the exclusion of higher risk groups earlier in pregnancy. Unfortunately the PNMR among the unbooked was much higher – 12 per 1000 (Chapter 8). The controls were matched to the probands and so they too will come from a lower risk background (Chapter 3). In consequence PNMR cannot be used as measures in this study to produce any useful conclusions amongst the booked women but comments are still valid. One woman who lost her baby said:

> We found the staff all cared for us with real thought and compassion in the most difficult of circumstances. Our main concern now is that we receive a full detailed account of what went wrong with the pregnancy. We hope no information will be withheld, and the truth will help us come to terms with our grief. This was to have been our first home birth having experienced three pretty awful hospital experiences previously. I was wonderfully relaxed and well in control of labour with breathing exercises alone. I would recommend a home birth to anybody.

Low birth weight

In the absence of the gold standard of PNMR, one turns to other criteria as measures of outcome. The proportion of babies born weighing under 2500 g was 0.6% in the home group, 1% in the hospital booked and delivered group and 2% in the home booked/hospital delivered group. All percentages are much lower than the approximate 7% of the total births in the UK. There were variations in the proportion of babies who were less than 37 weeks gestation; whereas 2% of the babies born to the home booked/hospital delivered group were delivered before 37 weeks gestation, only 1% and 0.3% respectively in the groups that were delivered in the planned place were delivered before that time.

A short-term measure of outcome may be assessed from the Apgar score and from resuscitation. The former is an undemanding measure of the baby's state; the latter reflects the professional's concern about the baby and his immediate post-delivery care (Table 6.2 and Figure 6.1). Examining the babies with an Apgar score below 7 at 1 and 5 min shows a trend. In Table 6.2 only 4% of babies home booked/home delivered were at this level at 1 min and 0.6% at 5 min. Among the hospital planned/hospital booked group these figures were 9% and 1% and in those

Table 6.1 Birthweight and gestation of babies reported by midwives (NBTF Home Births Survey 1994)

	Planned and delivered at home (*n* = 3922)		Planned and delivered in hospital (*n* = 3319)		Planned home but delivered in hospital (*n* = 769)	
	n	%	*n*	%	*n*	%
Birthweight						
≤2500 g	21	0.6	35	1.1	14	1.9
>2500 g	3738	99.4	3229	98.9	716	98.1
Not known/recorded	137		55		39	
p = 0.0007						
Gestation						
27–36 weeks	12	0.3	26	0.8	15	2.0
37–40 weeks	2810	72.6	2206	67.0	415	55.4
41–44 weeks	1048	27.1	1061	32.2	319	42.6
Not known/recorded	52		26		20	
p < 0.0001						

Table 6.2 Short-term measures of outcome reported by midwives (NBTF Home Births Study 1994); Apgar score < 7 at 1 and 5 min and babies receiving resuscitation

	Planned and delivered at home (*n* = 3922)		Planned and delivered in hospital (*n* = 3319)		Planned home but delivered in hospital (*n* = 769)	
	n	%	*n*	%	*n*	%
Apgar score < 7						
at 1 min *p* < 0.0001	157	4.1	308	9.3	89	12.1
at 5 min *p* = 0.0016	23	0.6	24	0.7	14	1.9
Resuscitation						
suction	364	9.3	596	18.0	165	21.5
bag and positive pressure	125	3.2	300	9.1	80	10.4
intubation	3	0.08	27	0.8	19	2.4
p < 0.0001						

who had home planned/hospital delivery were 12% and 2% respectively, showing a trend of increasing depression of respiration at birth in the three groups.

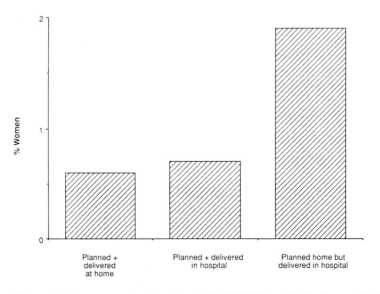

Figure 6.1 Apgar score less than 7 at 5 min (NBTF Home Births Survey 1994)

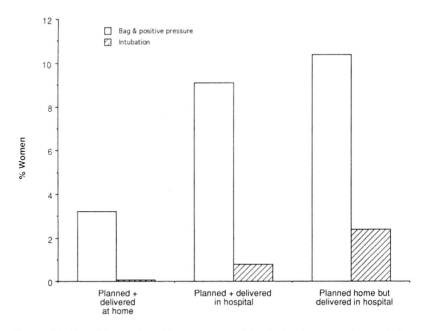

Figure 6.2 Use of bag and positive pressure and intubation in neonatal resuscitation (NBTF Home Births Survey 1994)

Table 6.3 Personnel performing resuscitation expressed as a percentage of babies having such treatment reported by midwives (NBTF Home Births Survey 1996)

Who resuscitated	Planned and delivered at home (n = 3922)		Planned and delivered in hospital (n = 3319)		Planned home but delivered in hospital (n = 769)	
	n	%	n	%	n	%
Midwife	375	89.3	451	53.2	73	33.3
Obstetrician	0	—	8	1.0	3	1.4
General practitioner	42	10.0	7	1.0	4	1.8
Paediatrician	3	0.7	339	41.5	136	62.1
Anaesthetist	0	—	6	0.7	2	—
Other	0	—	6	0.7	1	—

Looking at the data on the resuscitation methods used showed a similar picture (Figure 6.2). Whilst 13% of the home group received resuscitation, 28% of the hospital planned/hospital booked deliveries did, as did 34% of those home planned/hospital delivered, a steep increase.

The most intensive form of resuscitation is intubation, the passing of a tube through the larynx into the trachea and then giving oxygen under intermittent positive pressure. Only three of the babies home planned/ home delivered had this compared with 27 (1%) hospital planned/hospital delivered and 19 (2%) of those home planned/hospital delivered.

It is difficult to assess what constraint was placed on intubation by the lack of equipment carried by the midwife in the home and this is discussed later in this chapter. We did not perform this survey to examine the availability of resuscitation equipment in hospitals but in the 1984 National Birthday Trust Fund (NBTF) national survey on facilities available at the place of birth, all hospital units had at least one bag and mask; 523 of 528 reported they had intubation equipment. In that survey, (where only a few home births were assessed) in only 23% of deliveries at home was a neonatal laryngoscope available[1].

Modern resuscitation usage is reflected in Table 6.3 and Figure 6.3 which shows who did the resuscitation and should be read in conjunction with Table 6.2. It is seen that whilst 89% of resuscitation in the home was done by the midwife with 10% by the general practitioner (GP), of those who were home planned/hospital delivered, 62% of resuscitations were performed by paediatricians, 33% by midwives and very small numbers by obstetricians and anaesthetists. This emphasizes that paediatricians are readily available for the labour wards of hospitals to provide a speedy

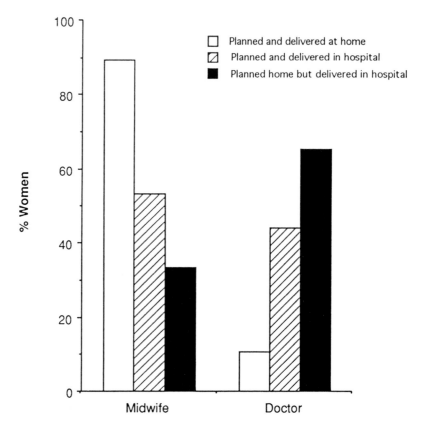

Figure 6.3 Personnel performing resuscitation expressed as a percentage of babies receiving such treatment (NBTF Home Births Survey 1994)

resuscitation. It also shows that the use of resuscitation of the newborn among those who were home planned/home delivered was low, especially for intubation. The use of the bag and positive pressure method which require simpler skills than intubation may well have been sufficient for this group. It is impossible to say further from a survey of this nature but a multidisciplinary working party of professionals is meeting at the moment on this matter and will probably give advice in the next months.

The position of the babies of the 769 women who had to be transferred to hospital is considered. The outcome for the baby was satisfactory in the vast majority of cases. Two of the stillbirths and two of the neonatal deaths occurred in women who intended home birth and transferred to hospital. None of the neonatal deaths were due to congenital abnormality. The last columns of Table 6.2 summarizes the incidence of Apgar score <7 at 1 and 5 min and the nature and extent of neonatal resuscitation required by this group of babies compared with those from the other main groups. It is impossible to state whether these differences reflect real differences in the condition of the baby at delivery or differences in practice related to location. However, the pattern of Apgar scores and of intervention is similar to that seen with maternal interventions, with the group transferred from home to hospital experiencing the highest rate of adverse outcomes.

There was only one set of twins born at home in this survey. The multiple pregnancy was diagnosed at 37 weeks gestation but the woman wanted to give birth at home as planned. Data relating to the labour came from the midwife only. It was reported that two midwives were present at the birth (38 weeks gestation) and the woman refused any form of examination. Twin 1 was a spontaneous vertex delivery with Apgar score of 9 at 1 minute and 10 at 5 min; twin 2 was a spontaneous breech delivery with Apgar score 4 at 1 min and 10 at 5 min. No problems were reported.

EQUIPMENT AVAILABLE FOR BIRTHS IN THE HOME

Examples of equipment available at a planned home birth were recorded in the questionnaire, including communication methods and resuscitation for both mother and baby. To assess what was available, we picked on certain sample items which might be needed in an emergency and that could not be sent on demand if an emergency suddenly arose, including some drugs and resuscitation equipment available at birth in case the mother or baby needed these immediately.

Oxygen and the necessary equipment to give intravenous fluids to the mother were available in just over half the births (Table 6.4 and Figure 6.4). The professional responsible for bringing these items to the house for the birth seems to vary around the country. In some areas, the midwife first-on-call for the birth, carries them; in others the second-on-call midwife goes to the local maternity unit to collect the necessary equipment while the first-on-call goes directly to the woman. In other areas, the GP is responsible for carrying some items. Problems arose when communication broke down between the professionals, when the labour proceeded so quickly that the baby was born before the equipment arrived or when the GP on call was unknown to the midwife so that she did not know which items were carried by the GP.

Table 6.4 Equipment available at the home birth – (for resuscitation of the mother) by regions reported by midwives (NBTF Home Births Survey 1994)

Region	*i.v. infusion set*		*i.v. fluids*		*Oxygen for mother*	
	n	%	*n*	%	*n*	%
Northern	62	56.4	60	54.5	75	68.2
Yorkshire	67	34.4	61	31.3	83	42.6
Trent	65	27.4	61	25.7	155	65.4
East Anglia	181	52.5	179	51.9	158	45.8
North West Thames	148	43.0	145	42.2	154	44.8
North East Thames	209	81.0	207	80.2	172	67.1
South East Thames	290	62.1	289	61.9	274	58.5
South West Thames	190	71.5	184	69.3	176	65.9
Wessex	154	59.0	152	58.2	97	37.7
Oxford	127	44.4	126	44.1	116	40.6
South Western	377	74.1	373	73.3	285	55.9
West Midlands	168	50.0	166	49.4	194	58.1
Mersey	31	29.5	30	29.2	29	28.3
North Western	61	25.6	57	23.9	93	39.1
Northern Ireland	13	54.2	14	56.5	23	95.7
Scotland	69	35.4	67	34.3	119	60.6
Wales	155	55.4	153	54.6	131	46.8
Not known/recorded Total 214						
Total UK	2367	53.2	2324	52.2	2334	52.4

One midwife commented:

> Sonicaid, entonox, bag and mask, narcan, oxygen were available for delivery, only that the midwife [responsible for] bringing them arrived after the delivery of the baby, owing to rapid delivery.

RESUSCITATION EQUIPMENT FOR THE MOTHER

Table 6.4 shows the basic equipment used for resuscitation of the mother if it proved necessary at a home birth.

We have commented elsewhere in Chapter 5 on how rarely serious sequelae such as postpartum haemorrhage occurred among the women booked for a home confinement. However, one does not know when such equipment will be needed in a hurry and so it is probably wise to have it available.

The presence of intravenous (i.v.) giving sets was reported in 53% nationwide with the highest proportions in North East Thames region (81%) where 258 women gave birth; South Western region (74% for 509

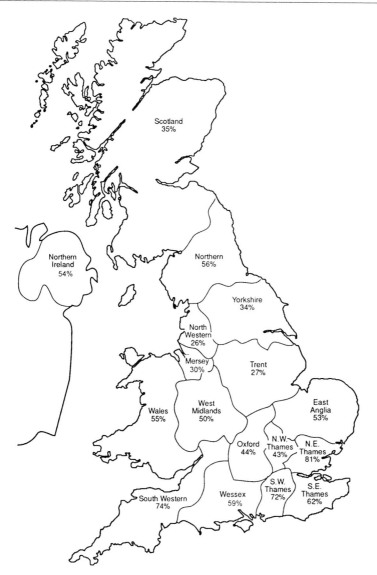

Figure 6.4 Intravenous infusion sets available at the home birth for resuscitation of the mother by regions (NBTF Home Births Survey 1994)

births) and the South West Thames region (72% for 267 births). Conversely in the Trent region, i.v. giving sets were only available for 27% of 237 births and in the North Western region 25% of 244 home births. Intravenous fluids mimic these data, being available at an average of 52% of home births overall with a similar regional distribution.

Some midwives carried intravenous infusion sets but admitted that they would be unable to use them if needed:

> We carry i.v. fluids but have no training in siting i.v.s. The equipment is carried so that it can be prepared for GP or paramedic crew. If we are to undertake home births more often, it is essential the midwife is able to site i.v. infusions. Our GPs do not carry equipment. The ambulance does.

Oxygen for the mother would have meant carrying heavy cylinders – even the portable ones weigh a lot when carried up a flight of stairs. Overall, only 52% of women in the UK had this facility at home births. The range of distribution is rather wider than the previous two pieces of equipment, ranging from 96% in Northern Ireland down to 28% in Mersey with 105 births. Since there were only 24 home births reported from Northern Ireland that means only one woman was without oxygen therapy but that 75 women in Mersey were without.

A comparison with data from a previous NBTF survey is given in Table 6.5 where the present survey is compared with one done by the NBTF 10 years before[1]. Although the numbers of home births in the 1984 study were small, it is very satisfactory to note the improved trend for all such maternal resuscitation equipment at booked domiciliary delivery from about a quarter to a half.

Similarly a sonicaid for easier detection of fetal heart sounds was present on 96% of home births' equipment compared with 88% in 1984. Such equipment is of great help and reassurance to midwife and mother.

In Table 6.5 are the reported communication systems. The telephone is a two-way system while the radiopager is mostly one-way bleeper only. The telephone availability is high at 93%, an increase on 1984 while the radiopager is about the same. In 1994, the average number of households with a telephone in England and Wales was 88% (ranging from 98% in social class I to 73% in social class V). Since the percentage of professional and non-manual families was higher in this study than nationally, then a higher rate of telephone availability is to be expected. Even so some 6% of home deliveries were without a telephone there.

Table 6.5 Equipment available at the home birth (NBTF Home Births Survey 1994 and NBTF Birthplace Survey 1984)

	i.v. infusion set for mother		*i.v. fluids for mother*		*Oxygen for mother*		*Telephone*		*Radiopager*	
	n	*%*	*n*	*%*	*n*	*%*	*n*	*%*	*n*	*%*
Total UK (Home Births 1994)	2367	53.2	2324	52.2	2334	52.4	4176	93.4	2587	57.8
Total UK (Birthplace 1984)	16	28.0	16	28.0	15	26.3	50	87.7	31	54.3

Had the midwives wished to summon aid, they would have had to send someone to a telephone which may have been distant.

> I had arranged for a second midwife to join me for the delivery but was unable to contact her when birth was imminent as no phone available.

Furthermore, a disturbing number of midwives reported breakdowns of their bleepers.

NEONATAL RESUSCITATION

Enquiry was similarly made into some sample items needed at neonatal resuscitation. Any professional who has assisted at a number of births has occasionally been faced with a newborn baby who unexpectedly does not establish a normal breathing pattern promptly and regularly. Minutes count and for such an emergency certain equipment should be there and the skills of the midwife/doctor present must be used for one cannot await help from a paediatrician. Hence all doctors and midwives who do practical obstetrics have been taught about standard methods of resuscitation of the newborn. Fortunately the needs are rare but practice is important. Skills are best kept by repeatedly performing a procedure – if a year or so goes by without needing to do a resuscitation obviously the practitioner will be less confident and less adroit. As well as these skills one needs certain equipment to perform emergency neonatal resuscitation and in Table 6.6 we analyse the results we obtained.

The most common item for neonatal resuscitation available at a home birth was the bag and mask (Table 6.6 and Figure 6.5); 6% of the midwives at home deliveries did not have this equipment, so that some 250 newborn babies did not have this available. This caused difficulties in some situations.

Table 6.6 Equipment and drugs available at the home birth for resuscitation of the newborn by regions reported by midwives. (1994 NBTF Home Births Survey)

Region	Neonatal narcan		Oxygen for baby		Bag and mask		Intubation	
	n	*%*	*n*	*%*	*n*	*%*	*n*	*%*
Northern	92	83.6	97	88.2	105	95.5	33	30.0
Yorkshire	124	63.6	186	95.4	176	90.3	51	26.2
Trent	211	89.0	231	97.5	226	95.4	43	18.1
East Anglia	271	78.6	227	65.8	334	96.8	74	21.4
North West Thames	172	50.0	289	84.0	324	94.5	136	39.5
North East Thames	188	73.3	246	95.3	246	95.3	158	61.2
South East Thames	265	56.7	437	93.4	454	97.2	303	64.7
South West Thames	192	72.3	258	97.0	249	93.6	137	51.7
Wessex	172	65.8	178	68.0	251	95.7	114	43.8
Oxford	156	54.5	270	94.4	258	90.2	107	37.4
South Western	295	57.8	428	84.1	494	97.1	159	31.4
West Midlands	265	79.0	319	95.5	308	91.9	84	25.1
Mersey	68	65.1	72	68.9	85	81.1	17	16.0
North Western	167	70.2	200	84.0	223	93.3	56	23.5
Northern Ireland	21	87.0	23	95.7	20	82.6	8	34.8
Scotland	143	72.7	164	83.3	184	93.4	43	21.2
Wales	199	71.1	247	88.2	248	88.6	61	21.8
Not known/recorded Total 214								
Total UK	3001	67.3	3872	86.8	4185	93.8	1584	36.3

When the baby was born he needed resuscitation (cord was tight round neck). Not having a bag and mask made resuscitation more difficult as all we had was an oxygen mask attached to oxygen cylinder. I feel very strongly that better infant resuscitation equipment is required for planned home births.

Narcan is a drug with the specific action of reversing neonatal depression caused by opiates given to the mother in labour for analgesia. This is most commonly pethidine but the drug can also act against morphine and heroin. Two-thirds of midwives (67%) reported carrying narcan, so that up to a third of midwives did not carry it; however if they did not offer pethidine or morphine as a method of pain relief in labour in the home this might be an explanation. The proportion of midwives with narcan dropped to 50% in North West Thames and was also low in Oxford, South East

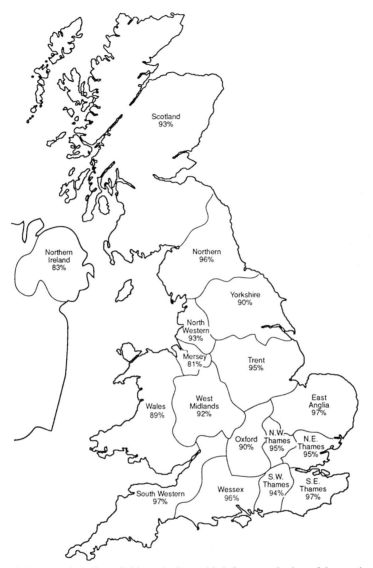

Figure 6.5 Bag and mask available at the home birth for resuscitation of the newborn by regions (NBTF Home Births Survey 1994)

Table 6.7 Equipment and drugs available at the home birth for resuscitation of the newborn. (NBTF Home Births Survey 1994 and NBTF Birthplace Survey 1984)

	Neonatal narcan		Oxygen for baby		Bag and mask		Intubation	
	n	%	n	%	n	%	n	%
Total UK (Home Births 1994)	3001	67.3	3872	86.8	4185	93.8	1584	36.3
Total UK (Birthplace 1984)	Not recorded		49	85.9	Not recorded		13	22.8

Thames and South Western. Compared with this over 80% had neonatal narcan available in the Northern, Trent and Northern Ireland regions.

Oxygen for the baby was available in 86.8% in the whole UK and in eight old regions the proportion was over 90%. However, in East Anglia, only 66% of home births have oxygen available for the baby, mirroring the low proportion of mothers (46%) who had access to this facility in that region.

Most babies born at home would be resuscitated by a close fitting face mask attached to an elasticated bag which allows manual positive pressure gas flow to the baby's lungs. Among 3896 home deliveries, 125 (3%) were resuscitated with a bag using positive pressure artificial respiration and this was done mostly by the midwife. Such equipment was available to 94% of home deliveries, 14 of the regions reporting over 90% coverage.

Even more rarely is intubation of the trachea used. We had no way of telling if this was an under use but we do know that there were 157 babies with Apgar scores below 7 in the home births group and 21 of them still had an Apgar of <7 at 5 min. Only three of 3896 home booked/home delivered babies were reported as being intubated; this compared with 27 of 3315 hospital booked/hospital delivered babies where 24 such babies had an Apgar score of <7 at 5 min. That number may be the effect of intubated resuscitation at 2–4 min so we cannot comment on the related needs of intubation by site of birth.

Again comparison was made with the NBTF 1984 study (Table 6.7). The availability of intubation equipment had risen from 23% to 36% but a survey like this could not examine the skills of the midwives and doctors present at birth and who may be called on to perform urgent neonatal resuscitation when the baby does not breathe.

Table 6.8 Birth injuries reported by midwives (NBTF Home Birth Survey 1994)

	Planned and delivered at home (n = 3922)		Planned and delivered in hospital (n = 3319)		Planned home but delivered in hospital (n = 769)	
	n	%	*n*	%	*n*	%
Bruising	13	0.3	47	1.4	16	2.1
Cephal haematoma	4	0.1	1	0.1	6	0.8
Caput succedaneum	6	0.2	12	0.4	8	1.1
Nerve palsy	2	—	1	0.1	1	—
Not known/recorded	30		13		24	

BIRTH INJURIES

Birth injuries were very rarely reported from any of the places of delivery in this study (Table 6.8). In the home planned/home delivered group, they amount to 1% of which bruising was by far the commonest. In the hospital planned/hospital delivered group it was 2%, again bruising dominating and the same picture was seen in the home planned/hospital delivered group where it amounted to 4%. Table 6.8 gives the details. We report these data for completeness.

MALFORMATIONS

The congenital abnormalities displayed in Table 6.9 are very important to the parents but of less value in assessing the nature of outcome of labour and its events; such anomalies had started in pregnancy many months before labour and do not reflect on the events of childbirth. There is no significant difference between the three groups of women delivering, talipes being the commonest abnormality in all groups. We report these data for completeness.

One mother whose first baby was born with a chromosomal abnormality remarked on the benefit she felt from giving birth at home:

> ...she was later found to have a chromosomal problem – the experience of the home birth was a major plus factor in what was a very dark time.

Table 6.9 Congenital abnormalities reported by midwives (NBTF Home Births Survey 1994)

	Planned and delivered at home (n = 3922)		Planned and delivered in hospital (n = 3319)		Planned home but delivered in hospital (n = 769)	
	n	%	n	%	n	%
Talipes	15	0.4	16	0.4	2	0.2
Cleft palate	8	0.2	5	0.2	1	0.1
Cardiac abnormalities	2	—	5	0.2	0	—
Hydrocoele	2	—	3	0.1	1	0.1
Dislocation of hip	2	—	3	0.1	2	0.2
Other	42	1.1	20	0.6	14	1.7
Not known/recorded	41		14		29	

INFANT FEEDING

Details about feeding the baby were obtained from the mothers' questionnaires and so again the totals will differ slightly from those of the midwife questionnaires. Questions were asked of the mother within 48 h of delivery and are dealt with in Tables 6.10 to 6.12. The 6-week follow-up study of a 20% sample of those mothers who took part in the study asked the same questions about feeding. Although the follow-up study was sent out at 6 weeks, some of the women filled in the questionnaires after this time; 89% of questionnaires returned in the follow-up study were within 9 weeks of delivery although the last went up to 17 weeks.

The proportion of breast-feeding in the first 48 h from the home booked/home delivered group was 80% compared with only 58% in the hospital delivered and 78% among those of the home booked/hospital delivered group.

This is confirmed in Table 6.11 as being the method of preferred feeding planned by the mother beforehand in over 90% in all cases. Conversely bottle feeding was carried out by 33% of the hospital booked/hospital delivered from the beginning (in 92% this was the planned method) compared with only 15% of the home booked/home delivered and 13% of the home booked/hospital delivered. Mixed feeding, always a harder method to establish, was planned and performed in less than 10%.

Table 6.10 Infant feeding within 48 h and at follow-up reported by women (NBTF Home Births Survey 1994)

	Planned and delivered at home		Planned and delivered in hospital		Planned home but delivered in hospital	
	n	%	*n*	%	*n*	%
Within 2 days	(*n* = 4191)		(*n* = 3470)		(*n* = 806)	
Breast only	3351	80.1	2008	58.1	628	78.5
Mixed breast and bottle	216	5.1	307	8.9	71	8.9
Bottle-feeding only	617	14.7	1142	33.0	101	12.6
Not known/not recorded	7	—	13	—	6	—
$p < 0.0001$						
Follow-up (see text)	(*n* = 721)		(*n* = 611)		(*n* = 132)	
Breast only	474	65.7	269	44.0	86	65.2
Mixed breast and bottle	76	10.5	74	12.1	16	12.1
Bottle-feeding only	155	21.5	257	42.1	29	22.0
Solids	16	2.2	11	1.8	1	0.8
$p < 0.0001$						

Table 6.11 Mother's wishes and baby's response to feeding in first 48 h reported by women (NBTF Home Births Survey 1994)

	Planned and delivered at home (*n* = 4191)		Planned and delivered in hospital (*n* = 3470)		Planned at home but delivered in hospital (*n* = 806)	
	n	%	*n*	%	*n*	%
Mother planned to feed this way	3988	95.7	3130	91.5	721	90.2
Not known/reported	25		50		7	
$p < 0.0001$						
Response of baby to first feed						
(More than one answer accepted)						
Fed well	3296	78.8	2513	72.9	622	77.9
Not interested	492	11.8	434	12.6	90	11.3
Sleepy	487	11.6	556	16.1	101	12.7
Irritable	36	0.9	71	2.1	17	2.1
Sick	90	2.2	103	3.0	17	2.1
Other comments	41	1.0	35	1.0	12	1.5
Not known/reported	7		9		8	
$p < 0.0001$						

Table 6.12 Regional analysis of women's wishes to breast-feed reported by women (NBTF Home Births Survey 1994)

Region	Planned and delivered at home		Planned and delivered in hospital		Planned home but delivered in hospital	
	n	%	*n*	%	*n*	%
Northern	102	98.1	105	96.3	31	96.9
Yorkshire	161	94.2	158	92.4	45	93.8
Trent	218	97.3	178	92.7	40	95.2
East Anglia	294	95.5	250	92.6	50	94.3
North West Thames	287	96.0	201	89.3	49	89.1
North East Thames	253	94.8	125	87.4	45	83.3
South East Thames	419	95.0	227	90.8	65	90.3
South West Thames	238	96.7	161	94.7	40	87.0
Wessex	249	96.1	156	94.5	37	94.9
Oxford	266	95.7	209	90.5	53	91.4
South Western	480	96.0	377	91.3	89	92.7
West Midlands	279	95.9	242	91.3	52	85.2
Mersey	103	97.2	69	86.3	17	100.0
North Western	218	95.2	173	93.5	29	80.6
Northern Ireland	21	95.5	21	95.5	1	100.0
Scotland	151	96.8	152	93.8	47	94.0
Wales	243	93.8	204	89.9	29	80.6

A regional analysis of how the mother planned to feed is seen in Table 6.12 and Figures 6.6 and 6.7. The home booked/home delivered group was consistently high and reflected the national average of 96%. The hospital booked/hospital delivered group had a somewhat lower average level (92%) with the lower limits of the range of 86% in Mersey. The home booked/hospital delivered group had an even wider range. Numbers of women were smaller than those in columns 1 and 2 but three regions were in the lower 80% level (North East Thames, North Western and Wales).

Further regional analyses were made of how the babies were actually fed in the first 48 h. This is interesting to compare with the mother's intent (Table 6.12) and with what was happening 6 weeks later (Table 6.10 is derived from answers to Q16A of the follow-up study). A reduction from expectations to actuality occurred in breast-feeding proportions in all regions among the home planned/home delivered group; this was about 15% in most regions but the reduction was over 20% in four – Northern, Yorkshire, Trent and Wales regions. The actual reduction of

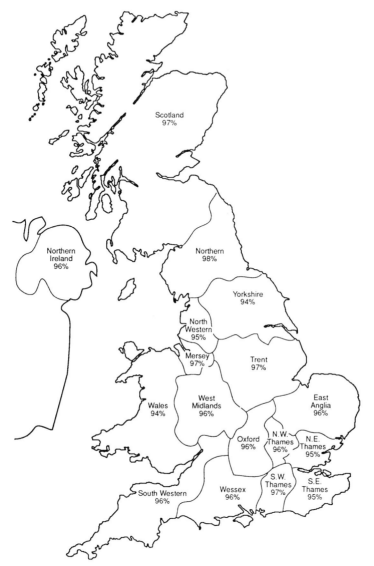

Figure 6.6 Regional analysis of women's wishes to breast-feed; planned home/ delivered home (NBTF Home Births Survey 1994)

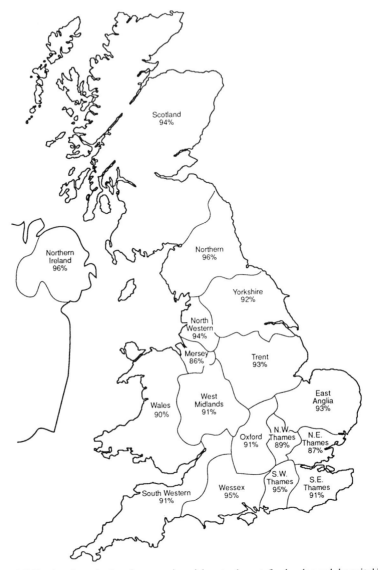

Figure 6.7 Regional analysis of women's wishes to breast-feed; planned hospital/ delivered hospital (NBTF Home Births Survey 1994)

breast-feeding was even more pronounced in the hospital booked/hospital delivered group, the greatest being in Northern, Mersey and North Western regions.

Assessing what was happening in the follow-up showed 65% to be still breast-feeding whereas the bottle feeding group had increased to 21% with 11% on mixed feeding (see Chapter 9). The data from this survey are higher than information about breast-feeding in some other studies[2–4], possibly due to the higher social class of participating women in the NBTF survey.

The mothers were asked how the first feed went. Fortunately, in all groups over three-quarters of the babies latched on well; just over 10% appeared not interested in each group and between 11% and 16% were said to be sleepy. Approximately 2% in the hospital delivered groups were irritable but only 1% in the home booked/home delivered group. Between 2% and 3% were sick and this is seen in all groups. Regional assessment showed a wide range but the individual numbers were not great enough to analyse any trend.

It would seem that three-quarters of babies settled on the planned feeding method and about a quarter were not interested or sleepy. We do not know when exactly this first feed was offered and it may be that the mother or the child were still under the effects of delivery, of analgesia given to the mother and transmitted transplacentally or even the effects of an operative procedure. It is important that the first feed is a happy one because much of the future feeding management depends upon this.

CONCLUSIONS

In a survey of 6000 births (with 4700 controls) among normal women, one would expect very low mortality rates. No maternal deaths and low perinatal mortality rates were reported among the booked women.

Reduced Apgar scores and perceived needs for resuscitation are other softer measures of outcome; here the home delivered babies needed or received less resuscitation. Equipment for intubation was available for about a third of home births while bag and mask was there in over 90% with 87% having oxygen for the baby. Birth injuries were rare and trauma rates low. Breast-feeding rates immediately after birth in the home deliveries were 80% and 58% in the hospital group. Six weeks later both were reduced (66% and 44% respectively). There was a slight regional variation, more in the hospital than the home group.

REFERENCES

1. Chamberlain, G. and Gunn, P. (1987). *Birthplace*. (Chichester: John Wiley)
2. Flint, C. (1993). *Midwifery Teams and Caseloads*. (Oxford: Butterworth-Heinemann)
3. Graffy, J.P. (1992). Mothers' attitudes to and experience of breast-feeding. *Br. J. Gen. Pract.*, **42**, 61–4
4. Murphy-Black, T. (1989). Midwives' role in postnatal care. *Nursing Times,* **85**, 54–5

7

Choice and satisfaction

CHOICE

Women taking part in the survey were asked about their decision to book a home delivery and the circumstances in which they made their choice. The major reasons given are shown in Table 7.1.

Choice of home births

Women choosing home birth did so for a variety of reasons, over 30% citing a desire for less interference as the main one:

> No drips, no stitches, no people walking in and out.

Twenty-five per cent of women found the convenience of home birth attractive;

> Being able to use my own lavatory without a nurse bursting in to make sure you haven't died.

Women planning home birth were more influenced by previous birth experiences than those who planned a hospital birth. They cited their previous experience of both home and hospital birth as a reason for choosing to deliver at home in 21% of cases.

> After spending eight days in hospital with my first baby I was allergic to the idea of sleepless nights and hospital routine.

Ten per cent of women choosing home birth did so because they were frightened of hospital birth. This fear of hospital birth related to a variety

Table 7.1 Main reason for choosing place of birth reported by women (NBTF Home Births Survey 1994)

Reason	Home		Hospital	
	n	%	*n*	%
Safety	0	—	2848	84
Less interference	1476	31	0	—
Convenient	1214	25	0	—
Previous home birth	481	10	2	0.1
Previous hospital birth	547	11	203	6
Frightened of hospitals	489	10	0	—
Continuity of care	217	4	0	—
Not known/recorded	239		103	

of factors – a hospital phobia since admission as a child, fear of the clinical environment, hospital rules and procedures.

Continuity of care was rated as the most important factor by 4% of women choosing home birth, while none of the women choosing hospital birth alluded to this.

> Because I opted for a home birth, I had my antenatal care from my community midwife, whom I have come to trust.

When the reasons for choosing home birth were analysed on a regional basis, the desires for less interference and for convenience were the two most commonly stated reasons. In three regions (Trent, East Anglia and Wales) convenience was the reason most commonly stated for wishing to have a home birth.

Choice of hospital births

Women who chose to give birth in hospital were almost unanimous in their reason for so doing. Over 80% cited safety as the reason for choosing hospital birth.

> I wanted the peace of mind of knowing that should anything be wrong with the baby or me immediate help would be available.

> Because we lived 45 minutes away from the hospital, we eventually decided to have the baby there. Our reason for doing this was that in the event of an emergency it would take too long to get there.

By contrast, safety was not mentioned by any of the women choosing home birth as a factor in making a decision about place of birth.

Timing of the decision

Women intending to give birth in hospital have usually made that decision before pregnancy (63%) or in early pregnancy (33%) while women choosing to deliver at home took longer to arrive at this point. Forty-one per cent of this group had decided before pregnancy and a further 39% during early pregnancy, leaving 20% still undecided by mid-pregnancy.

> I think for me the decision making was staged – I had always envisaged myself having a baby at home then when I was pregnant I thought I would, provided everything was okay, so I did not discuss it with GP/midwife/consultant until after my booking, bloods and scan, and then after that I never decided I WILL HAVE A HOME DELIVERY COME HELL OR HIGH WATER! – only that that was what I wanted as long as I continued to be normal. So there are two parts of the process – 'I want to if...' and 'asking professionals if I can'.

Who helped make a decision?

In keeping with the fact that the decision to deliver in hospital was usually made before conception or early in pregnancy is the lack of consideration given by these women to alternatives to hospital birth. Only 18% of this group considered an alternative place of birth. This may be due to the fact that they approached their doctors or midwives with the decision already made or may reflect a lack of discussion of options. Table 7.2 lists the options discussed with women planning hospital birth.

This indicates a disappointing lack of information about the options for choice of place of birth despite the aspirations of the Department of Health Expert Maternity Group[1] and The Royal College of Obstetricians response to the Changing Childbirth Report[2].

> Home birth is an acceptable option and appropriate information should be given[2].

Some women chose home birth because of lack of choice.

Table 7.2 Other options regarding place of birth reported by women planning hospital births (NBTF Home Births Survey 1994)

Option	n	%
Home birth	877	25
General practitioner unit	401	12
DOMINO	947	27
Other	41	1
Not known/recorded	58	

Table 7.3 Individuals with whom women discussed planned place of birth reported by women (NBTF Home Births Survey 1994)

Individual	Home		Hospital	
	n	%	n	%
Husband	4581	91	2826	81
Mother	3225	64	1060	30
Community midwife	3867	77	1393	40
General practitioner	3361	67	1052	30
Friends	3286	65	814	23
Not known/recorded	6		21	

> Hospitals and postnatal wards should be made more attractive so that there is a real choice. Also more DOMINO schemes so that going into hospital is not a big deal.

> If the DOMINO scheme had operated in our area I would probably not have had a home birth.

Women choosing to deliver at home were much more likely to discuss their plans with others (Table 7.3 and Figure 7.1).

Few women planning hospital birth were discouraged from this plan by those they talked to, while women planning home birth did so in the face of a certain amount of perceived discouragement.

> Why can't you be like ordinary women and go into hospital.

> Oh, aren't you brave.

However, general practitioners (GPs) were the only group who were perceived to be more likely to discourage than to encourage home birth (Table 7.4).

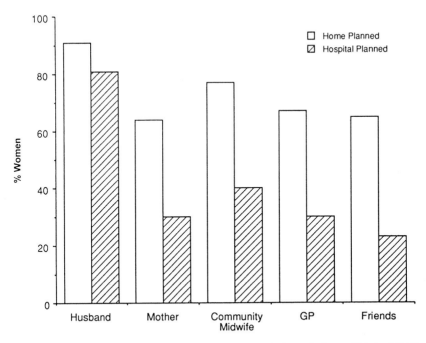

Figure 7.1 Individuals with whom women discussed planned place of birth (NBTF Home Births Survey 1994)

Table 7.4 Perceived response to planned home birth reported by women (NBTF Home Births Survey 1994)

Person	Encouragement		Discouragement	
	n	%	*n*	%
Husband	4217	85	384	8
Mother	2322	46	622	12
Community midwife	3595	72	219	4
General practitioner	1435	28	1665	33
Friends	2688	54	1124	22
Not known/recorded	6		6	

In a small number of cases, women were discouraged from home birth because of lack of GP cover (5%) and the woman's past obstetric history (5%). By far the most frequently cited reason for discouraging home birth was the lack of safety, which was cited as a reason for discouraging home birth in 53% of cases. Many women reported particularly vehement negative reactions from their GP:

I resent the way she tried to manipulate me and frighten me into a hospital birth.

A midwife, herself in her second pregnancy was told that she would run a high risk of having a brain-damaged baby if she delivered at home:

Doctors effectively washed their hands of me.

The doctors were looking for any excuse to get me into hospital.

A GP, married to a GP reported:

Most opposition and adverse comment was received from fellow members of the medical profession.

Discouraging comments from a GP included this pearl:

If I were a GP's wife he would divorce me!

Professional opposition to intended home birth may have unintended and unanticipated adverse effects. One woman reported that active discouragement from medical staff resulted in:

A hardening of my resolve to have the baby at home. This resulted in my holding out at home longer than perhaps I should have ... it seemed like the medical staff had triumphed ... I had to become entrenched to get what I wanted which made the mental shift necessary and what seemed like capitulation very difficult.

This seems a sad breakdown of communications.

Only 5% of women were discouraged from their planned hospital birth, by their friends or by their community midwife. The commonest reason stated was the increased obstetric interference associated with hospital birth. Once again, such opposition to the woman's plans can have unforeseen adverse effects.

My community midwife encouraged a home birth and I think she lost interest in me because I chose to go into hospital. Also I think she underestimated the skills of the hospital staff.

This woman's partner related:

On arriving at the hospital we were apprehensive as our midwife had caused us to be so.

The choice of birth place for any future birth is one way of assessing a woman's satisfaction with her choice (Table 7.5). The vast majority asked

Table 7.5 Choice of birthplace in the future reported by women (NBTF Home Births Study 1994)

Birthplace	Home		Hospital	
	n	%	*n*	%
Home	4704	94.7	152	4.4
Hospital	115	2.3	3105	89.3
GP unit	23	0.5	95	2.7
DOMINO	7	0.1	0	—
Midwife unit	4	—	0	—
Not sure/no choice	113	2.3	123	3.5
Not known/recorded	32		31	

to go back to the previous site and only 4% of those who planned hospital birth intended to deliver at home next time while 2% of those who planned home birth intended hospital birth next time. Some women in both groups indicated a wish to deliver in a GP unit next time. The closure of so many GP units deprives many women of this option.

SATISFACTION

In this section, the results of two groups of women are discussed: women who had planned a home delivery and women who planned to give birth in hospital.

The women had been asked to complete the questionnaire as soon as possible after the birth of their baby while the memory of their labour was still fresh in their minds. The majority were able to do this within 48 h and so we gained a picture of the satisfaction with the care they received, the good and bad aspects of the birth and the continuity of midwifery care.

Satisfaction with professional care

The majority of mothers in both groups reported that they were very happy about their decision regarding the place chosen to give birth to their babies. Table 7.6 shows that in the home group 98% of mothers were very happy and in the hospital group 90% were very happy with a further 9% feeling moderately happy.

The mothers were asked to describe how they felt about the care they had received from the midwives at their baby's birth. Table 7.7 and Figure

Table 7.6 How women felt about their choice of place of delivery by planned place of delivery (NBTF Home Births Survey 1994)

	Home planned		Hospital planned	
	n	%	*n*	%
Very happy	4719	98	3129	90
Moderately happy	88	2	303	9
Not very happy	7	< 1	19	< 1
Rather unhappy	6	< 1	12	< 1

p<0.0001

Table 7.7 Care from midwives at the birth reported by women (NBTF Home Births Survey 1994)

	Planned and delivered at home (*n* = 4191)		Planned and delivered in hospital (*n* = 3470)	
	n	%	*n*	%
Very satisfied	3915	94.3	3054	88.4
Satisfied	177	4.3	347	10.0
Dissatisfied	18	0.4	30	0.9
Very dissatisfied	11	0.3	9	0.3
Don't know	29	0.7	13	0.4
Not known/recorded	41		17	

7.2 show that almost all women in both groups were very satisfied or satisfied with their care.

Midwives can be pleased with achieving such positive results on the assessment of care they provided. One mother, who gave birth at home, even attached a gold star to the questionnaire to grade her high level of satisfaction. Many mothers illustrated their answers by commenting on just how satisfied they felt, for example:

> Local community midwife has been wonderful and a great support. Deserves a medal and should be canonized!!

Similar positive comments relating to good midwifery care were cited by the group who gave birth to their babies in hospital:

> I can only have good comments about the treatment that all the staff have given me. In particular all the lovely midwives who took care of me whilst in hospital up to and after the birth of my baby. I could not have wished for a better group of people.

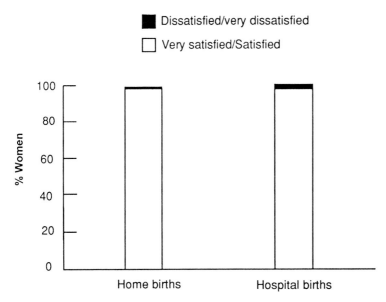

Figure 7.2 Satisfaction with care received from midwives at the birth (NBTF Home Births Survey 1994)

However, 29 women out of 4191 (1%) were less than satisfied with the midwifery care they had received at home, and a further 29 said they did not know how they felt. Thirty-nine women out of 3470 (1%) women were dissatisfied or very dissatisfied with their midwifery care in hospital and a further 13 could not decide how to rate the care. These 68 women make up a very small percentage of the total sample of the two subsets (1%), but it is important that they are not ignored and that their comments are noted.

The following two mothers described the dissatisfaction they felt with the care received from the midwives who attended them at home. In both cases, it appears that relationships between mother and midwife had broken down and they were now at odds as to how best to proceed, with the result that both mothers felt lack of support and loss of control. The first mother felt that her midwife became unreasonable by continuing the care at home when transfer to hospital seemed, according to her, inevitable:

> The midwife concerned was so into home births, she was determined for me to have it at home; she kept telling me to push when I did not feel like it and it was absolutely agonizing as the baby wasn't in the right position. Even when the ambulance was

Table 7.8 Care from midwives at birth (NBTF Pain Relief in Labour Follow-up Survey 1990)

	n	%
Very satisfied	858	75.4
Satisfied	223	19.6
Dissatisfied	32	2.8
Very dissatisfied	11	1.0
Don't know	14	1.2

> outside my house, she kept trying for me to push and was getting a bit cross with me.

The second mother also felt that her midwife had become uncaring – for very different reasons:

> Whilst my known midwife was technically competent, she was antipathetic about home birth. She was constantly anxious and obviously regarded the birth as an ordeal to which I was subjecting her. She spoke to me as though I were a naughty, imbecilic child.

Another mother, describing the unsatisfactory care she had received in hospital, wrote:

> I feel very upset at the midwife as she was too harsh and controlling.

She went on to explain why she felt this way. None of her wishes written in her birth plan had been granted and she compared this birth with a previous one, which also took place in hospital, when the midwives had been kind, understanding and had listened to her questions and requests.

Those data may be compared with the 1990 NBTF survey on Pain and its Relief in Labour[3] when women were asked the question about satisfaction with midwife care at the 6-week follow-up. The majority of births in that study took place in the hospital setting and therefore the findings should be compared with the hospital group in the 1994 study.

The women in the 1994 survey were also asked to rate the care received from their doctors at the birth of their baby (Table 7.9 and Figure 7.3). In the majority of cases, especially in the home birth group, this was not applicable since no doctor was present. If these cases are excluded, then it can be calculated that 93% of the home birth group and 94% of the hospital group were satisfied or very satisfied with their care. Some

Table 7.9 Care from doctors at the birth reported by women (NBTF Home Births Survey 1994)

	Home births (n = 4191)		Hospital births (n = 3470)	
	n	%	*n*	%
Very satisfied	859	68.4	1059	66.9
Satisfied	304	24.2	423	26.8
Dissatisfied	41	3.3	28	1.7
Very dissatisfied	32	2.5	12	0.7
Don't know	20	1.6	62	3.9
Not applicable	2835		1840	
Not known/recorded	100		46	

women reported on satisfaction with doctors' care in general although the question was specific to the birth.

As in the assessment of professional midwifery care, these are very encouraging results but here too there were women who were less than satisfied with the medical care they received – 73 women (6%) of the home birth group and 40 women (2%) in the hospital group. A total of 82 women could not decide how to assess the care they had received.

Perhaps the important feature the answers to these questions shows is that the satisfaction with medical and midwifery staff is high among the home and hospital delivered groups although among those who delivered at home doctor dissatisfaction was higher than in the hospital group.

Use of birth plans

A question on the use of birth plans was included in the midwives' questionnaires. In the home birth group, a little over one-third (36%) of the women had written one. Another 204 midwives had commented in one way or another that this task had not been necessary since a good relationship had developed between midwife and mother and a plan had been discussed verbally. Since the same midwife or small team of midwives would continue the care, then the mother's wishes were known by all and if the labour did not proceed according to plan, then the appropriate changes would be made with the agreement of the mother.

Even fewer women in the hospital group completed a written plan for labour – 903 women (28%). A further 150 midwives noted that a verbal

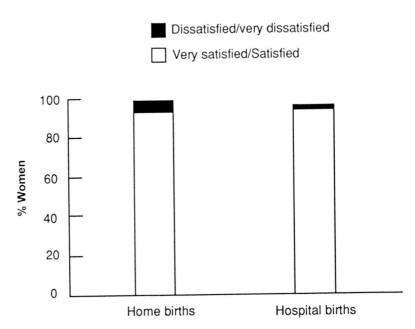

Figure 7.3 Satisfaction with care received from doctors at the birth (NBTF Home Births Survey 1994)

plan had been discussed either before labour commenced or on admission to the labour ward.

> Although I had not met either of my two midwives previously, I felt completely at ease with them and they took the time to read my birth plan and applied it throughout.

When the plan could not be followed, in 143 cases, the most common reason was a deviation from normal labour. Table 7.10 lists the reasons given.

Satisfaction with place of delivery

The mothers were asked to consider what they had liked most and least about having their baby at the place of their choice. The questions were open ended, but the coding was simple since only nine issues in either group were raised.

Table 7.10 Reason birth plan not followed reported by midwives (NBTF Home Births Survey 1994)

Reason	Planned and delivered at home (*n* = 104)		Planned and delivered in hospital (*n* = 140)	
	n	%	*n*	%
Changed mind	20	0.5	23	0.7
Labour changed	70	1.8	82	2.5
Staff shortage	2	—	8	0.2
Faulty equipment	0	—	3	0.1
Unreasonable request	4	0.1	3	0.1
Did not have time	8	0.2	21	0.6
Not known/recorded	26		72	

Home births

Tables 7.11 and 7.12 with Figures 7.4 and 7.5 relate to the home birth group considering what the women liked and disliked most about their births.

Almost a quarter of this group (>24%) commented on the fact that they felt less anxious and stressed by being able to enjoy all the advantages of giving birth at home – surrounded by familiar people and things, feeling more in control of the situation, more involved in decision-making. A study on home births conducted in 1993 in the Northern Region found that mothers chose the same issues – 'felt relaxed' and 'felt in control' being the most popular phrases to describe what they had liked about the home birth[4]. Others in this NBTF survey identified one of these advantages specifically as the main choice – being in own home (19%); being in control (16%); being with family (14%); freedom of choice (11%). Three hundred and thirty women said that the best factor was having a midwife at the birth who was already known to her; others were not so confirming. Care by a known midwife will be discussed further in the next section. Some women listed many things that they felt had been good about the birth, because they found it difficult to identify one factor above all others. One mother wrote very forcefully what could be a credo for all women who want a home birth strongly. Her factors were:

(1) Not being hassled into giving birth to another person's timetable.

(2) Not being patronised by some (male) doctor, who does not know what giving birth feels like.

(3) Not being wired up to those wretched monitors – which perpetuate anxiety.

(4) Being able to use aromatherapy, massage etc.

(5) Giving birth without the glare of bright lights and furnace of hospital heating.

(6) Being able to cuddle my new baby with my partner in my own bed.

There were a few things, however, which the women did not like about the birth at home. Table 7.12 shows that although the majority (65%) said there was nothing of note, 1393 women (35%) described something which they had not liked.

They wrote about feeling frightened that something would go wrong and the baby would be put at risk, either during the labour or in the early postnatal hours when the midwives had left the family on their own.

Many had not bargained for all the interruptions which occurred during labour at home – family and neighbours popping in, telephone calls, unexpected guests. One mother explained that the worst thing about giving birth at home was:

> When the window cleaner put his ladders up at the window just as I was at the pushing stage!

This has been known (outside this study) to happen at hospital births also.

Some complained about being expected to continue to run the home because they were there, whereas in hospital they would have been cared for by the staff and have had no housework or cooking to worry about. They appeared to have lost the feeling of importance which hospital admission brings to some women. Being at home signified a normal occurrence to their friends and family rather than an extraordinary event. One mother who gave birth to her baby in hospital wrote:

> Being in hospital also made me feel 'special'. I enjoyed being set apart from the outside world for a short time.

The mess which resulted from the birth 'blood on my new carpet' was unexpected and a source of distress to some women, to others was the lack of analgesia available. One comment was:

Table 7.11 What women liked most about their home birth reported by women (*n* = 4191) (NBTF Home Births Survey 1994)

	n	%
Feeling stress free	994	23.7
Being in own home	769	19.1
Being in control	648	16.1
Being with their family	578	14.4
Freedom of choice	440	10.9
Knowing the midwife	330	8.2
No travel	187	4.7
Everything	69	1.7
Knowing the doctor	3	—
Not known/recorded	173	

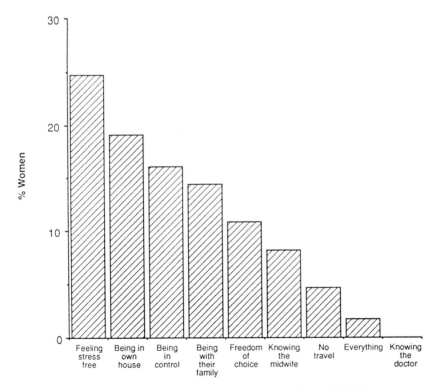

Figure 7.4 What women liked most about their home birth (NBTF Home Births Survey 1994)

Table 7.12 What women liked least about their home birth reported by women (*n* = 4191) (NBTF Home Births Survey 1994)

	n	%
Nothing	2573	64.9
Housework	259	6.5
Interruptions	255	6.4
Frightened something would go wrong	254	6.4
The mess	215	5.4
Lack of analgesia available	191	4.8
Midwifery care	181	4.6
Lack of information given	21	0.5
Transfer to hospital (after the birth)	17	0.4
Not known/recorded	225	

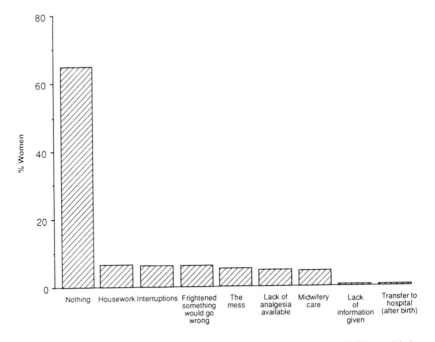

Figure 7.5 What women liked least about their home birth (NBTF Home Births Survey 1994)

There was no protective sheeting provided and nobody advised that we would need to supply our own. Our bed was ruined by waters breaking and blood at the birth. The gas and air ran out an hour before the birth and there was no back up supply.

In many cases, the second midwife-on-call brought the Entonox supply to the house after she had driven to the maternity unit to collect it. This could mean that the mother had to cope with the majority of the labour without the use of inhalational analgesia or may have already given birth before the arrival of the second midwife.

Hospital deliveries

The mothers' likes and dislikes relating to their stay in hospital are shown in Tables 7.13 and 7.14 with Figures 7.6 and 7.7. For more than half of the women (60%), safety was the most important factor. Many comments were written on this issue by both parents – the following are examples:

The discomforts of being in hospital are a small price to pay for the peace of mind of knowing that if anything goes wrong (as it did) the best possible care is available for both mother and baby.

I was extremely pleased that my wife was able to have our baby in hospital so that, if complications had developed, help was at hand.

The help and support available 24 h a day was appreciated by almost a third of the women (1009) – not just the technical assistance when problems arose but also the teaching and support received to enable her to care for herself and her baby. Some (131 mothers) even described their hospital stay as restful compared with home where they would have had to meet the needs of other young children, and a few (28) enjoyed the companionship and support of other postnatal mothers sharing their ward.

Like the home birth group, when they were asked to consider the thing they liked least about the hospital birth, a large number said that there was nothing of note (34%).

By far the biggest issue of complaint was the environment of the hospital (32%). This related to the postnatal areas, in the main, where the problems included the noise, the heat, the insecurity, the lack of facilities (baths, showers and bidets) and the food.

The only down-side of being in hospital is the constant activity night and day. Also the state of the toilets and bathrooms is

Table 7.13 What women liked most about their hospital birth reported by women (*n* = 3470) (NBTF Home Births Survey 1994)

	n	%
Felt safe	1984	59.7
Got lots of help	519	15.6
Nice, helpful midwives	490	14.7
Restful	131	3.9
Pain relief	80	2.4
No housework	51	1.5
Company of other mothers	28	0.8
The pool	24	0.7
Everything	18	0.5
Not known/recorded	145	

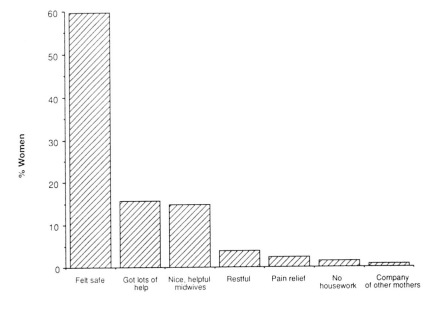

Figure 7.6 What women liked most about their hospital birth (NBTF Home Births Survey 1994)

Table 7.14 What women liked least about their hospital birth reported by women (*n* = 3470) (NBTF Home Births Survey 1994)

	n	%
Nothing	1066	34.3
Hospital environment	1011	32.4
Homesick	354	11.3
Hospital procedures	210	6.7
Inadequate staffing	207	6.6
Boredom, waiting around	128	4.1
Too many rules	113	3.6
Conflicting advice	26	0.8
Not known/recorded	355	

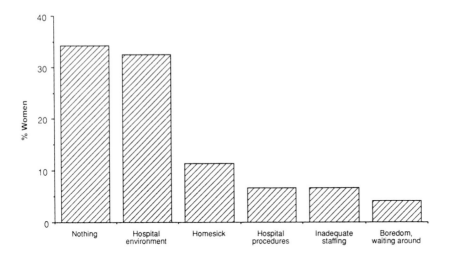

Figure 7.7 What women liked least about their hospital birth (NBTF Home Births Survey 1994)

disgraceful (plaster peeling off the walls), not conducive to relaxation or hygiene.

Postnatal experience is a lottery – it depends on whether the ward sister reveres routine or respects new mothers and their babies.

More than 200 women complained about the lack of help available due to insufficient numbers of staff on the postnatal wards. Many of them compared the wonderful one-to-one care provided by the midwives on the delivery suite with the hurried and inadequate care provided by the nurses on the postnatal wards. It is not clear from their comments whether the nurses they describe are nursing auxiliaries/health care assistants or whether they think that midwives in hospital assist women only during labour.

I was surprised, however, at the manner of the staff nurses on the ward. They didn't appear to be very caring and they were very noisy. The midwives, including the student, were very proficient and very geared to the needs of the delivering mother.

Some couples complained about the long wait experienced before they were allowed to go home from the postnatal wards. Often the reason for this was the policy for paediatricians to examine the baby prior to discharge and they were often delayed.

Known midwife

The mothers in both groups were asked whether they had a known midwife with them for labour and the birth of their baby. What was meant by known was not defined. It was possible therefore that women had received total care from this midwife over a long period of time or may have met her only briefly, e.g. at one visit in the antenatal clinic. She may even have had no care from her at all but only been introduced to her socially, e.g. at a coffee morning at a friend's house.

The group, therefore, who had noted that they had a known midwife with them at the birth were examined against other variables to determine when they met the midwife before or after the birth – in the pregnancy, during labour, transfer to hospital and repair of perineum. Table 7.15 shows the two groups of women who reported a known midwife with them at the birth and Table 7.16 shows the percentage of them who were cared for by her at other occasions reported by midwives. The wide difference of percentages shown in the home birth group reflect the

148

Table 7.15 The presence of the known midwife reported by women (NBTF Home Births Survey 1994)

	Home birth (n = 4191)		Hospital birth (n = 3470)	
	n	%	n	%
Present in labour	3470	83.0	1081	31.4
Present at birth	3495	84.0	1327	38.6

Table 7.16 Women with known midwife at birth reported by midwives (NBTF Home Births Study 1994)

Care given by known midwife, other than at the birth	Known midwife at home birth (n = 3495)		Known midwife at hospital birth (n = 1327)	
	n	%	n	%
Attended woman in pregnancy	2664	77.2	474	35.7
Attended woman in labour	3402	97.3	932	70.2
Repaired perineum	432	12.4	258	19.5

differing denominators (4191 compared with 3495). The actual number of known midwives reported at labour in the home are similar in each table (3470 and 3402, a difference of 68 in about 3400 (2.1%). In Table 7.16, the hospital group, the disparities are wider while 1081 women reported a known midwife was present in labour, 932 midwives concurred. These differences may reflect how well the women knew the midwife and the perceptions each side had of the relationship.

Many women who had chosen to give birth at home commented on the importance of knowing the midwife before labour. Some said that they had chosen home birth specifically so that they could ensure continuity of midwifery carer.

> I had to change my care *very* late in my pregnancy to a group practice because it was the *only* way I could guarantee to *know* the midwives who would be attending me as they have a caseload system.

> If I had another pregnancy, I think it would be a good idea to choose a home birth, even if I actually intend to have it in hospital in the end, just so that I could have the continuity of care of a known and trusted midwife.

In the hospital group less than a third (31%) had a known midwife with them in labour and not many more (39%) had a known midwife present for the birth. Table 7.16 shows the occurrence of a known midwife providing care in the two groups. These figures support the belief that women who give birth at home are more likely to know the midwife who attends them. Is this an advantage? Is this group more satisfied with the quality of midwifery care received? Only 8% of women having a home birth reported this as an advantage (Table 7.11). Perhaps it is a good idea but made more of by theorists than actual practice confirms.

Lee[5] states:

> Continuity of care is of no value unless the carer provides good quality of care.

In this NBTF study, the use of pain relief, the method of feeding, perineal damage, postnatal problems, the women's confidence and general feeling of contentment 6–8 weeks after the birth were examined to determine whether having a known midwife present at the birth made any difference.

There was very little difference between the two groups in relation to perineal damage. In the hospital group, women who did not have a known midwife with them at the birth had more chance of an episiotomy (15% compared to 10%). Surprisingly, no differences were found in the use of pain relief, the incidence of postnatal problems or the incidence in breast-feeding.

In both groups, more women were very satisfied with their care if this was provided by a midwife known to them (6% more in the home group and 8% more in the hospital group, see Table 7.17). However, the opposite occurs with the number of women who said that they were satisfied with the care received, so that when the two categories of very satisfied and satisfied are combined, there is very little difference between the group who had a known midwife present at the birth and the group who did not, whether the birth took place in the home or in the hospital (99.5% and 98% in the home; 99% and 99% in the hospital). Many comments were written by the mothers concerning the individual midwife, whether known to her or not:

> I was part of the new project whereby I had the same midwife/wives throughout my pregnancy, birth and postnatal care. I was *extremely* satisfied with this and consider myself lucky to have had this service. Despite not being able to have my home birth, the fact that I had my known midwife (who I knew and

Table 7.17 Satisfaction with midwifery care reported by women soon after birth (NBTF Home Births Survey 1994)

	Home birth				Hospital birth			
	Known midwife ($n = 3466$)		Other midwife ($n = 558$)		Known midwife ($n = 1272$)		Other midwife ($n = 1815$)	
	n	%	n	%	n	%	n	%
Very satisfied	3328	96.0	499	89.7	1189	93.5	1560	86.0
Satisfied	120	3.5	47	8.5	73	5.7	229	12.6
Dissatisfied	10	0.3	5	0.9	5	0.4	15	0.8
Very dissatisfied	4	0.1	2	0.4	2	0.2	5	0.3
Don't know	4	0.1	3	0.5	3	0.2	6	0.3

trusted) made the whole rather traumatic birth in hospital much easier.

For some, the presence of a midwife whom she knew and trusted was extremely important, with the result that if this was planned and expected but did not occur then the mother felt let down and unable to cope:

> I was dismayed to find (at 40 weeks) that one of my booked midwives was to be off work for several weeks due to family problems. Whilst I have sympathy for my midwife's problems, I do feel that where a home birth service exists more of an effort should be made to *guarantee* you are attended by your own midwife at delivery.

Such guarantees can never be given honestly so long as one group of human beings looks after other human beings. Midwives have their own lives to lead. Forty-three women who gave birth at home, reported that they had a known midwife with them for the labour but not for the actual birth. Similarly, 102 women who gave birth in hospital, had a change of midwife in the midst of labour.

> My first midwife changed shifts about 40 minutes before I gave birth. I found this very upsetting. A feeling of being deserted as though my baby was not important to her. I know she was tired but a week later I am still sad about it.

For others, although they had hoped to have their named midwife with them, this had not been possible but they were very happy with the care received:

> The midwife who attended me was not a midwife I had met during my antenatal care (I had met five). Initially I was concerned about this, but in the event it did not matter.

Continuity of care was an unexpected bonus for some women in the hospital group. Since previous births, teams of midwives had been introduced into their locality where each team takes responsibility for a finite caseload of women and each woman has a named midwife within that team. They described the improvement in care which this had brought and compared it to the previous fragmented care provided in the past by different midwives and doctors at every visit:

> After a particularly traumatic labour first time round, the continuity of care and being delivered by a midwife I had met made the second labour a much more manageable experience. I cannot praise the DOMINO scheme highly enough – and the security of hospital facilities and the privacy of birth attended by a known person.

Obviously to some who commented the issue of the known midwife was an important one, but satisfaction for the majority did not rest on this. In the home births with a known midwife 99.5% were satisfied or very satisfied with events but so were 98% who did not have a known midwife.

CONCLUSIONS

The choices made by the women in this study, their reasons for making these choices and the process by which they arrive at their decision, emphasize just how different are the two groups of women selecting home or hospital for delivery. Despite the fact that this study took place after the publication of the Changing Childbirth Report[1] and the professional bodies' response to it, there is little to indicate that either group had ready access to unbiased information about the options available, or that the decision about place of birth was an informed choice made after exploring all options. This can be partly excused by the lack of good quality information about outcome in relation to place of birth[6].

Great satisfaction was reported by both hospital and home birth groups but the latter had a slightly higher level than the former generally. A useful analysis of the reasons for choosing the site of booking may help planners. Midwife care seemed high and the few causes for dissatisfaction are considered. Medical care, less frequent at home deliveries, scored highly also but obviously impinged less on the mothers' thoughts.

Although professional care was well thought of, postnatal facilities in hospital did not satisfy the women so much.

REFERENCES

1. Department of Health Expert Maternity Group. (1993). *Changing Childbirth.* (London: HMSO)
2. Royal College of Obstetricians and Gynaecologists. (1994). *The Future of the Maternity Services,* p. 298. (London: RCOG Press)
3. Chamberlain, G., Wraight, W. and Steer, P. (1993). *Pain and its Relief in Labour.* (London: Churchill Livingstone)
4. Northern and Yorkshire Regional Health Authority. (1994). *Report of the Northern Region Home Birth Survey 1993*
5. Lee, G. (1994). A reassuring familiar face. *MIDIRS Midwif. Dig.,* Sept. **4**(3), 277–9
6. Young, G. (1996). Should there be a trial of home versus hospital delivery in the United Kingdom? Uncertainty is likely to persist, but some knowledge is better than none. *Br. Med. J.,* **312**, 755–6

8

Home births not registered in the study

It had been the intent of the National Birthday Trust Fund (NBTF) Home Births Study Team to examine booked home births only, for it was considered that the most valid data would come from looking at the management and outcome of births in the sites that had been planned. The main survey concerned those who by 37 weeks gestation had intended to and booked to deliver at home and their controls with similar intents for hospital delivery. Those with unplanned home births obviously could not be similarly invited to join a survey prospectively and so might introduce bias. There are, however, a large number of home births that are unbooked, as many as 40% in some studies. The NBTF enquiry therefore was extended to get some basic objective information about those women who delivered at home, unplanned or unbooked. The two adjectives describe two different populations: the former, a much larger group, might have booked at a hospital but not managed to get there in time; it could, however, also include some women who had always intended to deliver at home despite their apparent booking cover. The latter group may have included some who were still late in pregnancy considering booking at hospital, general practitioner (GP) Unit, or for a home delivery but the baby had come unexpectedly before they had fulfilled their plans; there would also be many who never intended to go to hospital or receive antenatal care.

Requests were made to the Supervisors of Midwives to list those women who had had babies delivered at home but were unbooked for domiciliary delivery. A simple questionnaire was sent to the Supervisors of Midwives which asked about delivery, attendants, outcome and any transportation to hospital (Appendix). We could not get full information from women and delivering midwives for it was considered this would be impossible to do. Even more important would be the lack of registration prospectively (37 weeks in the main study) and so bias could be introduced.

There were 1600 women reported in this unbooked group during the year, making about one-fifth of all the home births examined in this study (5971 + 1600 = 7571). Their distribution varied in the regions of the country as shown in Table 8.1 and Figure 8.1. Wales, Scotland and West Midlands reported among the highest proportions (over 10%) whilst the South East of England reported lower proportions of unbooked deliveries at home. The lowest of all was Northern Ireland with less than 1% – ten women compared with the reported 24 who had booked domiciliary confinements.

Table 8.2 shows the proportions of survey-reported booked and unbooked home births. The unbooked made up a considerable proportion, being over 30% in seven of the regions, rising to 55% and 45% respectively in Scotland and the Northern Regions. Even the lowest reported rates in South West Thames and South Western Regions were 14% and 16%.

There was one set of twins born in this group. The mother was aware that she was carrying twins and was booked for a hospital birth. However, labour commenced at 39 weeks gestation while she was visiting friends and proceeded too quickly for transfer. Two midwives were present at the births – one baby cephalic, the other breech. Both babies and mother were well but all were transferred into hospital for observation since the mother had a history of postpartum haemorrhage.

Among those who had an unplanned home birth, 1445 (91%) reported that they had in fact booked at a hospital but did not make it there. Another 67 (4%) had booked for a home birth; of these, 26 did not book until late pregnancy because, although they wanted to give birth at home, they felt they would meet opposition to this with their obstetrical histories or less than satisfactory home conditions.

> ...she lived in a bender [a simple tent supported by the bent branch of a tree] in the woods... preferred no medical aid... called midwife when she was in labour.

> This woman had a great deal of pressure put on her by GP to deliver in hospital. Both the midwife and the woman were unhappy with this and the delivery was straightforward.

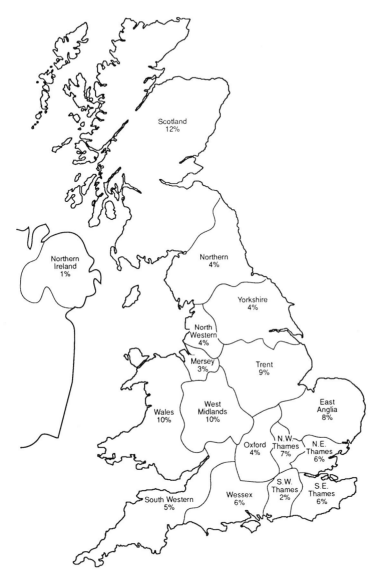

Figure 8.1 Unbooked births delivering at home by region (NBTF Home Births Survey 1994)

Table 8.1 Unbooked births by Region reported by Supervisors of Midwives, percentage of 1600 unbooked births (NBTF Home Births Survey 1994)

Region	n	%
Northern	70	4.4
Yorkshire	58	3.6
Trent	148	9.3
East Anglia	133	8.3
North West Thames	105	6.6
North East Thames	89	5.6
South East Thames	88	5.5
South West Thames	38	2.4
Wessex	93	5.8
Oxford	60	3.8
South Western	85	5.3
West Midlands	161	10.1
Mersey	51	3.2
North Western	58	3.6
Northern Ireland	10	0.6
Scotland	192	12.0
Wales	161	10.1

The remaining 41 were not registered in the study because they booked too late, because they moved home and delivered in a home which was not the planned one or because the midwife omitted to invite them to participate. Another 86 had not booked anywhere, the commonest reason for this was among 56 (4% of all) who had a concealed birth; in 14 (1%) the pregnancy had not been diagnosed, ten of whom reported that they did not know about the baby until they were in labour.

Those 1445 women who had booked in hospital may have included many who had gone through a booking process and either changed their mind late or had no intention of delivering there. This is seen in the comments for example:

> This lady booked for a hospital confinement early in her pregnancy and because her last baby delivered rapidly she decided to have a home confinement at 39 weeks.

> Patient daughter of Community Midwife. She was booked for hospital but it appears she intended to be delivered by her mother at home. Therefore did not call her mother until in advanced labour.

Table 8.2 The regional distribution of home births planned and unplanned reported by midwives (NBTF Home Births Survey 1994); derived from Tables 4.1 and 8.1

Region	Home births (n)			% Unbooked of total
	Booked	Unbooked	Total	
Northern	88	70	158	44.3
Yorkshire	162	58	220	26.4
Trent	202	148	350	42.2
East Anglia	316	133	449	29.6
North West Thames	304	105	409	25.7
North East Thames	229	89	318	28.0
South East Thames	414	88	502	17.5
South West Thames	235	38	273	14.0
Wessex	241	93	334	27.8
Oxford	251	60	311	19.3
South Western	445	85	530	16.0
West Midlands	295	161	456	35.3
Mersey	96	51	147	34.8
North Western	217	58	275	21.0
Northern Ireland	23	10	33	30.3
Scotland	158	192	350	54.8
Wales	246	161	407	39.4
Total	3922	1600	5522	29.0

The 34 women booked for hospital and delivered at home are not included for reasons given in the text

PARITY

Among the 1600 women, in 19 instances there were no data on parity. For the rest, 233 were primiparous (15%). About 85% were multiparous and 101 were grande multiparous (6%) having had at least four babies before.

GESTATIONAL AGE

Supervisors of Midwives reported data about gestational age for 1519 while in 81 could not complete this information; four babies were born before 24 weeks, the remainder are distributed in an exponential curve which reached an apex at 40 weeks with a decline sharply afterwards. (Figure 8.2). The percentage of babies born before 37 weeks was 7%. These compare approximately with national data.

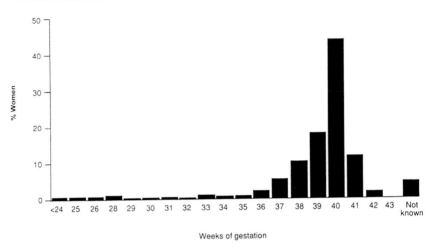

Figure 8.2 Unbooked births delivering at home by gestation in weeks (NBTF Home Births Survey 19994)

REASON FOR THE UNPLANNED HOME BIRTH

By far the commonest reason given for the unplanned home birth was a quick labour, given by 1250, 80% of the 1600 births reported. Among these, only 6% were primigravidae. Other reasons were preterm labour (4%) and concealed pregnancy (4%). This reason was given by 16% of the primigravidae compared with 2% of the multigravidae; 66 women (4%) refused admission. We have no way of going back on those refusals for this was a confidential enquiry and so we do not know at what point the suggestion was made by the midwife or GP for the move into hospital. In this group 59 were multigravidae and only seven were primigravidae.

Some 65 women (4%) gave a late decision about booking plans as a reason and ten women were unaware of being in labour, not surprisingly for they were in the group of 14 who were unbooked since they did not know they were even pregnant.

DELIVERY

In 227 cases (14%) it was reported that the woman was alone when she delivered (Table 8.2). Three-quarters of these (174) had a quick labour and 33 were concealed, 15% of those giving birth were alone compared with only 0.2% among booked home deliveries.

Deliveries before 37 weeks were 18%, compared with 7% in booked home births. The numbers were too small to allow firm conclusions but eight of the 20 babies who died in the unbooked group (five stillbirths and three neonatal deaths) were born to mothers who delivered alone, three times the expected number and allowing for small numbers, equivalent to a perinatal mortality rate of 35 per thousand. Two-thirds of these mothers and babies (68%) were transferred to hospital after delivery with the same proportions of reasons expected as in the whole group of unbooked births.

In another 202 cases (13%) the husband performed the delivery and he was present in a further 807 occasions (49%). A neighbour delivered the baby in 1%, a family member in 4%, a friend in 1%. In 775 cases (49%) a midwife delivered, whilst on 58 occasions (4%) this was by the GP while a family doctor was present in 115 cases (7%). An ambulance officer delivered on 216 occasions (14%). Amongst the other people present were a student midwife in 41 (3%) who went with one of the community midwives as part of the training process. The same could not be said for the 12 children of the family who were reported as being present, the two social workers or the four police officers.

TRANSFER TO HOSPITAL

In 652 instances (41%) both the mother and baby who delivered at home with no booking plans were transferred to hospital; in another three the mother only or in nine the baby only were transferred. This was done mostly by ambulance accompanied by a paramedic (37%), a midwife (31%) or both (23%). The obstetrical flying squad was responsible for the transfer of 20 women and the neonatal squad for ten babies, so that only 21 of the 65 women (13%) travelled without professional help. Motor cars were used on 12 occasions and a helicopter once. It is of interest and, in an anonymous survey is a bare fact only, that one woman was transferred to hospital by public transport.

The reasons for transfer were reported; the commonest was suturing of a laceration of the perineum or an episiotomy in 256 women (39%). This seems a high number when those who should be skilled enough to suture the perineum were available at the home in over half the cases. Others needed an intravenous infusion (3% of those transferred), blood transfusion was given to eight women and a manual removal of placenta took place in 21. In all, 46 women, including the 21 who had a formal manual removal, needed help with delivery of the placenta in the hospital. Only three women were reported as going to hospital to accompany the baby who had to go in and in two cases the reason given was the baby was to be

Table 8.3 Who delivered the unbooked woman reported by Supervisors of Midwives
(NBTF Home Births Survey 1994)

Who delivered	n	%
Midwife	775	49.0
GP	58	3.7
Obstetrician	3	0.2
Ambulance officer	216	13.6
Husband	202	12.7
Other family member	60	3.8
Neighbour	21	1.4
Other friend	9	0.6
Other	10	0.7
Not known	19	1.3
Woman was alone	227	14.3
Total	1600	100.0

adopted so the mother had to go to hospital. This seems a strange need for transfer and smacks of administrative convenience.

Enquiry about the reason for the baby being admitted was most commonly that the infant required incubator care in 125 instances (19%) with specific respiratory support in 37 (6%). Surgery was deemed the reason in only five instances. Warmth was specifically mentioned in 43 (7%); 62 babies (10%) were admitted for an examination. Without knowing details it is not possible to assess if such assessments could have been done by community paediatricians or at the outpatients' department in a few days time.

OUTCOME

We received data about livebirths, stillbirths and neonatal deaths but not about early neonatal deaths hence a true perinatal mortality rate cannot be given. Among the 1600 women there were ten stillbirths and ten neonatal deaths giving rates just above background: 6.3 per 1000 in each case; stillbirth rates nationally are about 5 per 1000 and early neonatal death rates are slightly lower than that. The comparative figures in this survey among home deliveries that were booked are 0.4 and 0.6 per thousand respectively, ten times less, but it must be remembered that these are small figures and the variation within such data does not allow any statistical conclusions. While the death rates were not significantly higher than background, stillbirth and neonatal death rates were much higher than in the booked home delivery group, information that confirms previous reports[1].

CONCLUSIONS

These data seem to under-represent the true picture. In previous years, the unbooked home births made up about 30% of all domiciliary births[1]. A more recent but smaller national sample was in the 1984 NBTF survey which confirmed this proportion[2]. There are no reliable national data available on booked/unbooked home deliveries following the inconsistencies of the national and regional maternity data collection systems refered to previously[3]. In our study they are 29% with the highest returns in Scotland (55%) and Northern (44%). A lack of previous contact with a midwife, more scanty records, poor outcome, or just exasperation of the midwife with her workload may have contributed. However, the returns to the brief questionnaire on unplanned home births came from the Supervisors of Midwives who should be aware of all deliveries in their area. On past experience one might expect about 70% of the home deliveries to be booked (about 8650) and 30% unbooked (about 3700). Why then did we get only 43% of the returns that might have been expected in the unbooked group (1600 of 3700) when in the booked group data return was 67% (4228 of 8650)? Possibly the Supervisors were overloaded with little support for data collection.

Another hypothesis must be considered in the absence of information about the true national proportions of booked/unbooked home births in 1994. Perhaps the increase in home births is mostly in the booked sector so our 5971 returns from booked home births are among 9000–10 000 planned home births (i.e. about 60%) and the 1600 reports of unplanned home births are among the 20% of the national 12 352 births (2470). With these national ratios, returns in this survey would be 60% for planned and 65% for unplanned. These must all be hypotheses in the absence of a properly run maternity statistical service, not even delegated to Regional Health Authorities but to overstretched District Health Authorities and Trusts.

Four-fifths of the unbooked deliveries we could comment upon reported that they did not have time to get to the place of booked delivery. Primiparous mothers made up only 6% of this group but about 40% of all women now having babies are primiparous. A larger proportion of those caught short in this study were multiparous. If the lapse was a genuine accident, there may be a place for better antenatal education to remind these women of the signs of onset of labour, and the way labour can progress insidiously and with speed in those who have had a baby before.

In about half the cases of unbooked delivery (49%) a midwife was there and did the delivery. In another 18% of occasions, a trained professional delivered although they may not have been trained in domiciliary obstetrics. Almost three-quarters of these unbooked mothers had some professional assistance. The real problem was with the approximately 20% who had a friend or family member only in attendance. For both mother and attender the experience must have been mind shattering. A sadder and more potentially dangerous situation were the 227 women who delivered alone.

From anecdotal evidence of women and midwives, an unknown proportion of this group included those who had gone through the motions of booking a hospital delivery to please their family, their GP and their midwife, knowing in their hearts that they intended to deliver at home come what may. One woman's comment recorded by the Supervisor of Midwives read:

> In order to get the home birth, I found myself in the quite ridiculous situation of lying to my GP to ensure that I got it which I found awkward and should not have been necessary.

To gain the trust of such women would be an important step so that support can be offered at a level which is non-pejorative and is not seen to be regimental. How far society should go to identify or reason with these potential mothers is a philosophical point much of which depends on the attitude of the professional concerned about the desirability of home delivery overall or, more specifically, unplanned home delivery.

From society's point of view, the economics of providing an emergency service to such a large group must be examined in these days of National Health Service financial auditing.

REFERENCES

1. Campbell, R., Davies, I.M., Macfarlane, A. and Beral, V. (1984). Home births in England and Wales, 1979. *Br. Med. J.*, **289**, 721–4
2. Chamberlain, G. and Gunn, P. (1987). *Birthplace.* (Chichester: John Wiley)
3. Campbell, R. and Macfarlane, A. (1994). *Where to be Born?* (Oxford: National Perinatal Epidemiology Unit)

9

The follow-up survey

Ann Oakley

Like many other aspects of childbirth, feelings about the place of birth may change with time. As mothers reflect on the meaning of what has happened, the experiences and circumstances surrounding the delivery may be seen in a different light. To this mediation of experience by time, may be added the impact on mothers and babies of what actually *did* happen, whether at home or hospital.

This chapter looks at the responses of a subsample of the study women to a postal questionnaire sent to them when their babies were 6 weeks old. The questionnaires went to a random 20% of the original sample who had agreed to be involved. The response rates (with no reminder letters) were strikingly high: 84% of the women in the planned home delivery group and 86% of those planning hospital deliveries. These figures indicate an impressive willingness on the part of the new mothers who volunteered to join the original survey to share their experiences with researchers, and in this respect confirm the findings of many other studies[1].

THE WOMEN RESPONDING

A total of 855 women who had planned home deliveries and 645 who had planned to have their babies in hospital returned the questionnaire. The mean age of the babies when the follow-up questionnaires were completed was 7.2 weeks for the home sample and 6.8 weeks for the hospital sample. In the event, 132 of the women who had planned home deliveries actually delivered in hospital (18%), and seven of those intending to give birth in hospital had their babies at home, similar proportions to the main study. As noted in Chapter 3, the subgroup of the home sample who delivered in hospital were significantly different from the rest of the group in terms of parity, with 38% of the home group who went into hospital having their first babies, compared to 11% of the home group who stayed at home. In some of the analyses the group intending to have home deliveries is separated into subsamples of those actually delivered at home and those actually delivered in hospital; the number of the actual home deliveries in the hospital booked group is too small to analyse separately. Tables are based on numbers answering particular questions.

Table 9.1 shows socio-demographic data for the women returning the follow-up questionnaires compared to the original sample. In the original sample, the women who planned home deliveries were significantly older, more highly educated and more likely to be middle class than those planning hospital deliveries. Most of the follow-up responders were white, middle class, and having their first or second babies, as were those in the main study. There were significant differences in parity, class and education between the home and hospital samples at the follow-up: more of those planning to have babies at home were having second or subsequent babies, had left education after the age of 16 and more were middle class according to partner's occupation. There were no significant differences in these variables between the original and follow-up samples for either planned home or planned hospital subsamples.

THE FOLLOW-UP SURVEY

The women answered questions about their memories of labour and delivery and about the early postnatal weeks in the follow-up questionnaire; in addition, two-thirds of the women and their partners provided detailed comments. Partners were enthusiastic contributors.

A considerably higher proportion of women in the home sample offered comments, possibly reflecting the greater controversy which continues to surround home birth (Table 9.2).

LABOUR AND BIRTH IN RETROSPECT

Three of the questions in the follow-up survey asked women to reflect whether they had enjoyed the birth of their babies, how much control of the labour they felt, and how much pain they experienced. The answers they provided to these questions are shown in Table 9.3.

It is clear that enjoyment of birth is more common with a home delivery: 95% of those who had their babies at home said they enjoyed the

Table 9.1 Characteristics of the follow-up survey responders compared with the original sample (NBTF Home Births Survey 1994)

	Main study				Follow-up survey			
	Planned home		Planned hospital		Planned home		Planned hospital	
	n	%	n	%	n	%	n	%
Age (years)								
≤29	1853	38	1433	42	305	37	242	39
30–39	2900	59	1931	57	506	61	371	60
40–49	138	3	56	1	21	2	9	1
			$p<0.0001$					
Parity								
0	791	16	553	16	139	16	100	16
1	1948	39	1620	46	325	38	302	47
2	1474	30	962	28	260	31	183	29
3 or more	773	15	364	10	129	15	56	8
	$p<0.0001$				$p<0.0005$			
Ethnicity								
White	4886	98	3447	98	837	98	636	99
Other	106	2	54	2	14	2	4	1
Social class (woman's occupation)*								
Middle class I, II & IIInm	3284	83	2237	78	584	83	438	82
Working class IIIm, IV, V	672	17	634	22	121	17	98	18
			$p<0.0001$					
Social class (man's occupation)†:								
Middle class I, II & IIInm	2816	62	1666	51	502	64	305	51
Working class IIIm, IV, V	1745	38	1621	49	287	36	298	49
			$p<0.0001$				$p<0.0001$	
Age of finishing fulltime education (years)								
≤16	1872	38	1775	51	313	37	323	51
17 or more	3112	62	1720	49	537	63	315	49
			$p<0.0001$				$p<0.0001$	

*Omits housewife and armed forces
†Omits unemployed, not applicable and armed forces

Table 9.2 Additional comments on follow-up questionnaires by place of delivery $p < 0.0001$ between columns 1 and 2 (NBTF Home Births Survey 1994)

	Planned home/ delivered home		*Planned hospital/ delivered hospital*		*Planned home/ delivered hospital*	
	n	*%*	*n*	*%*	*n*	*%*
Women	522	72	317	49	100	76
Partners	215	30	32	5	24	18

Table 9.3 Enjoyment, control and pain at birth in follow-up study by place of delivery (NBTF Home Births Survey 1994)

	Planned home/ delivered home		*Planned hospital/ delivered hospital*		*Planned home/ delivered hospital*		
	n	*%*	*n*	*%*	*n*	*%*	
Enjoyed birth	686	95	487	76	77	58	$p < 0.0001$
Completely in control during labour	446	62	187	29	29	22	$p < 0.0001$
No/very little pain	103	14	52	8	12	9	$p < 0.05$

birth, compared to 76% of the hospital sample. Not surprisingly, enjoyment of the birth was lowest (58%) in the group who had planned to have their babies at home but gave birth in hospital. The figures for the experiences of control in labour and of pain follow broadly the same pattern. The highest incidence of control is in the home-delivering group (62%), and the lowest in the group transferred to hospital (22%). While 14% of mothers having their babies at home reported no or very little pain, this figure was 8% in the hospital sample, possibly a reflection of the type of woman delivering in the home setting (Chapter 4).

There were no women in the home-delivering group who said they had felt not in control. Overall, the reported figures for control and enjoyment were 44% and 83%, respectively. These figures are substantially higher than comparable ones in a similar follow-up to a national sample of women studied in a survey of pain relief in labour[2], where 67% of women said they enjoyed the birth and 19% felt completely in control. This may reflect the target group for the survey which was volunteers among women who had planned to have a home delivery.

These issues of enjoyment, pain and control are linked in the additional comments written on the questionnaires. One mother spoke for many when she wrote:

I had complete trust in my midwife and if I do have any more children I would definitely have a home birth. I felt also that although labour was very painful (naturally) it was easier to bear knowing I was in control and because I was much more relaxed at home than in hospital. I was also surrounded by people who knew me and cared about me.

However, one mother who had a hospital birth regretted the modern emphasis on control, which might be interpreted as being independent of drugs or guidance:

There seems to be more and more stress on mothers 'being in control' during labour but this is being interpreted too often as a labour without drugs, e.g. my NCT antenatal class for my first child (I have had two children). Consequently, I had a dreadful experience first time – relying only on gas and air when I know now I would have benefitted from an epidural... Also, 'being in control' is not always a good thing during labour as it is quite reassuring for someone to guide you through it when you are feeling a lot of pain.

CHOICE AND DECISION-MAKING

The issues of choice, information and decision-making in maternity care have been highlighted in a 1993 policy document *Changing Childbirth*[3], and by a long tradition of user group involvement in the maternity care scene in the UK[4]. In these respects, the women in the follow-up survey confirmed many of the conclusions of previous research, whilst stressing more modern concerns about changes in childbirth policy and the impact of the new National Health Service (NHS) on maternity care provision.

The importance of choice was stressed by many women and their partners:

Women should be given a real choice of where to give birth. My GP assumed I would give birth in hospital and did not advise me of my right to have my baby at home.

But the emphasis on hospital birth means that parents may have to work quite hard to find out about other options:

I felt that I had to find out for myself how to book a home birth and what it involved.

As several parents commented, the availability of choice as to place of delivery may differ greatly from one area of the country to another:

> What concerns me is that when speaking with other women who live in other areas of the UK they are strongly discouraged or even refused *choice* when it comes to home birth, also in some hospitals.

In this respect, the maternity services clearly have a good way to go, as many comments made clear:

> On the whole, the midwifery service is excellent; however, doctors still tend to treat women as half-wits who do not need to be informed of their rights regarding *their* pregnancy, labour and subsequent birth experience. I felt as if I had to fight the whole time to be treated as an intelligent, informed human being.

Many women stressed the potentially key role the GP plays in the decision about place of birth. One commented that:

> As a GP is usually the first point of call for most women when they become pregnant, I feel it should be up to the GPs to be offering women choice as to where they can give birth and encouraging women to feel confident to, for example, choose a home birth as there is no evidence as yet to show that home is any less safe than hospital!

Another mother, a GP herself, found it interesting to reflect on her own experience of hospital delivery:

> Having had my next two children at home, I would like to see that opportunity more available everywhere to women...I think there is a long way to go with the relationship between midwives and GPs in particular and there needs to be more open discussion and trust as well as a real desire to look at the facts honestly. Unfortunately GPs now are so overloaded in every area of work that this may not happen easily.

Surveys of satisfaction with maternity care show a general bias towards declaring satisfaction with the choices that have been made, even though some aspects of the experiences lived through might have been less than satisfactory[1,5,6]. The percentages of women in both home and hospital samples who reported in the main study that they had made the right choice, were exactly the same; 96% said they had, 2% that the choice had not been the right one, and 2% did not know. Interestingly the figures,

Table 9.4 How women felt about their choice of place of delivery in main and follow-up survey, by planned place of delivery (NBTF Home Births Survey 1994)

| | *Main study* | | | | *Follow-up study* | | | |
| | *Home planned* | | *Hospital planned* | | *Home planned* | | *Hospital planned* | |
	n	*%*	*n*	*%*	*n*	*%*	*n*	*%*
Very happy	4719	98	3129	90	817	99	569	90
Moderately happy	88	2	303	9	7	1	60	10
Not very happy	7	<1	19	<1	0	—	2	<1
Rather unhappy	6	<1	12	<1	1	<1	1	<1
							$p < 0.0001$	

however, for the two groups were different in the follow-up questionnaire; as Table 9.4 shows, the women giving birth at home were more likely to say they were very happy about the choice they had made.

The women's answers to an open-ended question about why they felt either happy or unhappy about where their babies had been born showed that the most common single answer in the home group was that they valued the choice they had made (43%), whereas in the hospital group it was that they thought hospital was the safest place (53%). In the home group, 17% (none in the hospital group) valued the family involvement that was possible, and 11% (less than 1% in the hospital group) the fact they had control.

Confidence, support and territory are all related in women's accounts of the decision to have a home birth:

> ...as soon as I decided to have a home confinement I felt much more confident about the birth. This was due to the support from the community midwives – to be visited in your own home made me feel much more comfortable and relaxed about pregnancy/ labour.

When a baby is born at home, it is much easier for birth to be experienced as a family event. One father summed up the advantages of home birth thus:

> Home birth is obviously the most sensible way to deliver the child for the following reasons:
> Birth is not an illness.
> The experience at home is very moving for both partners.

The process is under the parents' control and not the consultant's.
It is far cheaper.
I recommend you look at the Dutch model.

Birth settings were not expected to be perfect. Those women planning delivery in hospital were aware of disadvantages such as separation from families and subjection to hospital regimes. However, far fewer women in the home birth sample mentioned disadvantages of their chosen place of delivery. There were, however, a few observations about the disadvantages of home birth. These ranged from the minor:

> ...so much equipment is needed to be brought into the home and the entonox is not always available in the required quantities. The small cylinders when full only last one hour.

to the more substantial:

> ...my midwife was sick from the EDD and so I had an on-call one. The birth was 1 hour 40 minutes and felt that on the whole she wanted it over as soon as possible. She ruptured my membranes, without discussion, gave the syntometrine injection immediately. Baby was not given to me immediately and cord was cut without waiting for it to stop pulsating as I would have liked. I then fed the baby and the midwife left, leaving me with a naked, grizzly baby, myself unwashed, unfed, and really not in control of the situation.

Most of the negative comments about home birth concerned the after-care. For example, one mother wrote that:

> In this area the midwife is excellent but I do feel that you are very much on your own after that. It would be nice to have some help in initial weeks with housework and younger children – tends to be friends/family who do this – not sure if that is a good or bad thing...

Both in the main and the follow-up questionnaires, women were asked where they would choose to have a subsequent baby. Here again there was a tendency to select the option that has already been experienced; more than 90% of both samples at both time points would choose the same place of birth again (Table 9.5 and Figure 9.1). But there are also differences, and women who had chosen a home delivery were significantly more likely than those who had chosen to have their babies in hospital to choose the same option again. Other research has shown a similar pattern[5,7].

Table 9.5 Women's responses about the next birth, immediately after birth and at follow-up, by planned place of delivery (NBTF Home Births Survey 1994)

	Main study				Follow-up study			
	Home planned		Hospital planned		Home planned		Hospital planned	
	n	%	n	%	n	%	n	%
Home	4704	95	152	4	820	96	39	6
Hospital	115	2	3105	89	20	2	556	87
GP Unit	23	—	95	3	12	1	47	7
					$p < 0.0001$			
Would choose same*	4704	94	3200	95	820	96	603	94
Would choose different	138	2	152	4	32	4	39	6
					$p < 0.05$			

* GP unit counted as hospital

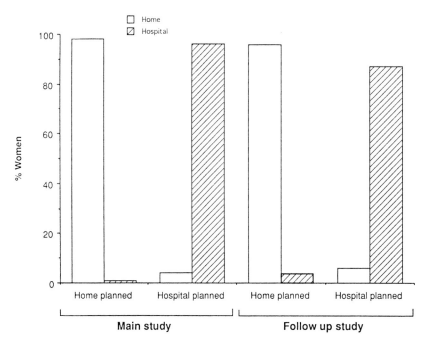

Figure 9.1 Women's responses about where to have the next birth; responses immediately after birth (main study) and at follow-up, 6 weeks later showing very little change (NBTF Home Births Survey 1994)

MOTHERS' AND BABIES' HEALTH

A series of questions were asked in the follow-up survey about mothers' and babies' health in the period since the birth. Some mothers and babies had been (re)admitted to hospital: 4% and 3% of mothers and 4% and 5% of babies in the home and hospital delivered groups respectively (these differences are not statistically significant).

Table 9.6 gives the figures for the two groups in both the post-birth and follow-up questionnaires for eight health problems which commonly feature in mothers' accounts of their health after childbirth. For all problems recorded in the post-birth questionnaire except for stress incontinence, the incidence was higher in the hospital group, and significantly so for tiredness, backache, headache and painful stitches. This pattern was intensified in the follow-up, with the incidence of all health problems except for stress incontinence significantly higher in the hospital group. The *absolute* levels of some problems recorded at the follow-up were striking: for example, more than two-thirds of mothers recorded tiredness, nearly a third backache, one in five headache and constipation, and one in four piles and tearfulness. These figures confirm the conclusions of the study by MacArthur and colleagues[8] that there are significant levels of physical morbidity after childbirth, with many symptoms going unrecorded and untreated.

Unsurprisingly, perhaps, the figures for the home planned group in Table 9.6 conceal rather different fates for the women intending to deliver at home who actually did so and those who actually delivered in hospital. The incidence of all the health problems was significantly higher in the hospital-delivered subgroup, with statistically significant differences for backache (21% and 33%), constipation (15% and 24%), stress incontinence (5% and 14%), painful stitches (6% and 30%), piles (21% and 34%) and tearfulness (21% and 33%).

Women having hospital deliveries were more likely to receive treatment for their health problems. There may be links between this and some of the negative comments women made about the quality of postnatal care following a home delivery.

When it comes to mothers' emotional well-being, there are clear differences between those having a hospital and a home delivery (Table 9.7). Both feelings of high cultural well-being and confidence as a mother are more common among women intending to have their babies at home who actually did so, compared to women experiencing a hospital delivery, and lowest when this was not intended. These figures for feeling very

Table 9.6 Health problems post-birth and at follow-up by planned place of delivery (NBTF Home Births Survey 1994)

| | Main study | | | | Follow-up study | | | |
| | *Home planned* | | *Hospital planned* | | *Home planned* | | *Hospital planned* | |
	n	*%*	*n*	*%*	*n*	*%*	*n*	*%*
Tiredness	590	69	479	74	556	65	458	71
			$p<0.05$				$p<0.05$	
Backache	297	35	279	43	192	22	194	30
			$p<0.001$				$p<0.001$	
Headache	66	8	73	11	135	16	138	21
			$p<0.05$				$p<0.01$	
Constipation	90	11	86	13	140	16	147	23
							$p<0.005$	
Piles	117	14	110	17	196	23	201	31
			$p<0.0005$					
Painful stitches	97	11	162	25	81	10	111	17
			$p<0.0001$				$p<0.0001$	
Stress incontinence	41	5	30	5	54	6	56	9
Tearfulness	128	15	117	18	197	23	183	28
							$p<0.05$	

happy and very confident as a mother in this sample are 50% and 40%, which compare favourably with figures of 37% and 21% in the follow-up to a national study of pain relief in labour[2].

Table 9.8 shows infant feeding by place of delivery: 44% of the mothers delivering in hospital were still breast-feeding by the time of the follow-up survey, compared with 66% of those planning home delivery who had their babies at home, and 65% of the women who planned home delivery but had their babies in hospital. Figures 9.2 and 9.3 show the same data, by whether the woman knew the midwife, reinforcing the finding from other parts of the survey that the known midwife made little difference to the feeding patterns or their variations at 6 weeks.

The women's comments suggest that more help with breast-feeding is usual following a home delivery:

> Felt that the problems I experienced with 'latching' on with breast-feeding were handled [in a] more relaxed [way] compared to

Table 9.7 Emotional well-being in follow-up study by place of delivery (NBTF Home Births Survey 1994)

	Planned home/ delivered home		Planned hospital/ delivered hospital		Planned home/ delivered hospital	
	n	%	*n*	%	*n*	%
Feeling now						
Very happy	362	50	261	40	54	41
Happy	318	44	332	52	62	47
Quite/very depressed	26	4	39	6	12	9
Don't know	15	2	13	2	4	3
$p < 0.0001$						
Confident as a mother						
Very	246	34	150	23	28	21
Quite	470	65	480	75	101	77
Not very/not at all	6	<1	14	2	2	2
Don't know	1	—	0	—	1	<1
$p < 0.0001$						

Table 9.8 Baby feeding in follow-up study by place of delivery (NBTF Home Births Survey 1994)

	Planned home/ delivered home		Planned hospital/ delivered hospital		Planned home/ delivered hospital	
	n	%	*n*	%	*n*	%
Breast	475	66	284	44	86	65
Bottle	156	22	273	42	29	22
Both/other	92	13	88	14	17	13
$p < 0.0001$						

the care I received in comparison with my previous hospital deliveries. Midwives are contactable 24 hours a day which is very reassuring and Mums are made to feel that they *should* contact... as and when necessary. [Home birth].

One thing I get depressed about...is the fact that I desperately wanted to breast-feed my baby. I did the first feed after the birth (when I was told two different ways by two different midwives). Then once on the ward, *no one* talked to me about breast-feeding. I felt so alone! I gave up the first night as I and my baby got very upset because I could not latch the baby on properly. I admit I never asked for help in the hospital but they all seemed so busy and I think they maybe should have noticed that overnight I had

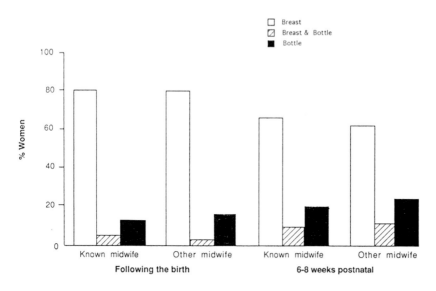

Figure 9.2 Methods of infant feeding among women delivering at home with known or unknown midwife (NBTF Home Births Survey 1994)

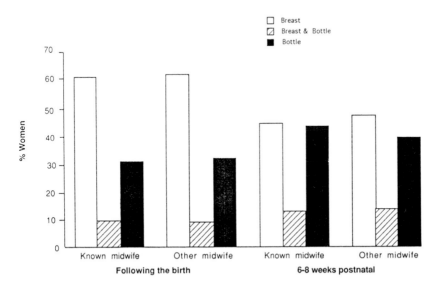

Figure 9.3 Methods of infant feeding among women delivering in hospital with known or unknown midwife (NBTF Home Births Survey 1994)

changed from breast to bottle. I just wish now that I had shouted out for a lot more help! [Hospital birth].

DISCUSSION

The voluntary comments give great insight into how the experiences and responses of women planning home deliveries differed from those of women planning to give birth in hospital. Women booked for home deliveries talked about the problems of negotiating this, with unco-operative GPs and hospital doctors figuring prominently in their comments; they complained about the difficulty of even knowing that home birth was an option. They stressed the advantages of home births in terms of relaxation, control and avoidance of unnecessary intervention, and praised midwifery care. They drew attention to the need for better postnatal care, especially for first-time mothers, and commented on the problem of the handover in care from the midwifery team to health visitors, which often seems irrational from the viewpoint of both mother and baby. In the hospital group, the most frequent themes were perceived safety but also inadequate, inappropriate and stressful antenatal care; poor postnatal care, including much conflicting advice, and stays that were too short for the mother to get enough rest and learn enough about taking care of her baby.

Trying to get a home birth

Like many previous surveys, the comments women and their partners made on this subject portray home birth as still being an unpopular option among health professionals, and one which consequently has to be fought for by parents who want it[9-11]. Many women contrasted the theoretical right women may have to a home birth with what happens in practice:

> More support is needed from medical professionals, (i.e. consultants/GPs) for women who wish to have their babies at home. I found that I was strongly discouraged by the hospital consultant in particular from having my baby at home. Perhaps more research (such as yours) into home birth would help to allay their fears.

Assertive was a word used by many women:

...As I am a young mother (only 19 when I had my first child), I feel that you have to be very assertive with all health officials when it comes to where and how you want your baby.

The crucial role of GPs in the negotiation process came in for a lot of criticism, as noted earlier. Some GPs had not only discouraged the option of home birth, but had been more deliberately obstructive, as in this woman's experiences:

...One thing which will always stick in my mind... is that I was an unwanted patient after I told my GP I wanted a home birth. I think GPs attitudes towards home births should change. Being pregnant is not a disease but a sign of good health and giving birth at home is only a natural thing to do.

Underlying much of the debate about home birth are different perceptions of risk. More than half the women planning to have their babies in hospital took the view that birth in hospital is safer. Sometimes the opposition to a mother's right to choose home birth explicitly mentions issues of risk and safety:

Many would have liked a home birth but we have frightened people into thinking hospital is the only safe place! I felt nervous and cautious before but now I feel it was entirely normal, as indeed it was normal procedure for all our grandparents in both families.

One mother, herself a statistician, noted that interpreting risks is an exercise that also involves preferences:

I was surprised at how strong I had to be to have a home delivery. I felt that GPs' and consultants' opinion that I should deliver in hospital, based on the statistical probability that I may haemorrhage (PPH 500 ml with my first baby), did not take account of the fact that I am a responsible educated person (and also a statistician) to whom the risks can be explained. Without the support of a midwife who took account of me as a person and my preferences, I would probably have dutifully trotted off to hospital.

The mother may have understood the role of risk taking better than many others because of her professional knowledge. She deserved an impartial discussion of what the risks of a repeat postpartum haemorrhage might be.

Hospital maternity care

Some of the women's comments on postnatal care confirm the findings of other research identifying this as an area which needs much improvement:

> All I needed after the birth was a shower in a clean warm bathroom and lots of tea to drink. Neither was available in hospital when I wanted them. There was not very much support in the hospital after the birth. I was left very much to myself, no one came to tell me how to change a nappy or how to bring wind up. I was not counselled on breast-feeding or given any support, encouragement or practical advice on how to latch on my baby.

Early discharge emerged as an issue about which many women expressed strong opinions:

> It is now the trend for mothers to go home within 48 hours. I had long labours with both my children and felt very tired for weeks afterwards (also breast-feeding). I feel that although *no* pressure was put on me to leave hospital, we should be *encouraged* to stay in as long as possible, especially when we have other children waiting at home!

Although women in the two groups had different observations about the experience of birth in different settings, there were also impressive similarities in the themes in both the hospital delivered and home delivered women's comments:

(1) They expressed the need for informed choice;

(2) They stressed the importance of continuity of care, not only during labour and birth but from pregnancy through the postnatal period;

(3) They emphasized the midwife's role;

(4) They voiced disquiet about current changes in the NHS, including cost-cutting exercises that might be to the detriment of mothers and babies.

Continuity of care

The major theme from the comments women and their partners made in the follow-up survey was the importance of continuity of care. The value of seeing the same midwife throughout pregnancy was explained simply by one woman thus:

> I think if you see the same midwife during your pregnancy you come to trust her and feel like you have a friend coming to help you out for the birth. It makes it all so much more relaxed as all your questions have been answered and this person knows how you want things to go as you will have talked over everything beforehand. It makes you feel much more confident about the whole thing yourself, therefore helping to ensure things go well.

The importance of continuity of care may often be stressed as an ideal from which practice falls short and the need for continuity in order to avoid conflicting advice was particularly stressed, and especially for first-time mothers:

> In hospital post-delivery, I wish there was more help and encouragement with breast-feeding. Each time I asked for help, I was attended by a different nurse/midwife giving conflicting advice... On discharge home I was attended by four different midwives over 6 days, again all giving conflicting advice.

Many of the views expressed confirm the need for the postnatal care given by midwives to be more geared to mothers' needs. In this, as in other respects, the follow-up data repeat the findings of other surveys of maternity care. An earlier study of postnatal community midwife care, for example, found that 22% of mothers complained of inconvenient or rushed visits; 14% wanted more help than was given, and 13% wanted more information and/or demonstration of care. Fragmentation of care was identified as a particular problem[12].

The women in the follow-up survey offered many comments about failures to ensure continuity of care in the postnatal period:

> With regard to receiving visits from your midwife 10 days after the birth of your baby, these visits were carried out but nearly every day a different midwife visited; I only saw my own midwife the once. I felt this gave no consistency whatsoever and would have preferred to see the same midwife over the period of the 10 days.

Health visitors came in for a healthy amount of criticism – a finding borne out by other studies[13]:

When it came to health visitors, if they are all the same as mine they are a waste of time. She always looks for problems and does not believe that anyone might enjoy having a new baby to care for (even if it does render you brain dead after a week). She is totally unreliable, does not turn up when expected and then talks total tripe when she does appear.

The solution to these problems ensuring continuity of care adopted by some parents was to pay for the care of independent midwives. One woman stated the logic behind her decision in no uncertain terms:

I had to pay an independent midwife to get the cover I needed or wanted. My GP does provide services for home birth but could not guarantee a midwife that I knew would deliver my baby. The reason for choosing a home birth was familiarity/developing a relationship with the person delivering my baby. To end up with a stranger delivering my baby would not have been acceptable.

This may have been an extreme point of view but it reflected what others wanted. Some mothers recognized that there had been real attempts in some areas to move towards team midwifery:

Team midwives are the best thing that has happened; they take good care of you. If you cannot go to the doctors for your check they will come out to you. When you go into labour or if you are worried about anything, they come out to you in a matter of 10–15 minutes. Excellent service.

The role of the midwives

Just as continuity of care is prized as an ideal, so the personal care provided by midwives is regarded as the lynchpin of a good maternity service. This holds true irrespective of place of birth:

I think midwifery is a brilliant profession and all those I have met during the pregnancy deserve medals for their dedication, skill and enthusiasm. Well done!

The midwives became my friends. They helped me to realize that having a baby was the most natural thing in the world. I always thought that women who said they enjoyed giving birth were mad, but this time I can honestly say I agree with them – and it's down to the midwives.

Satisfaction with care from doctors and midwives was not asked about directly in the follow-up questionnaire. When asked about this in the main questionnaire, satisfaction with midwifery care was much higher than satisfaction with the care provided by doctors, but far fewer women in the subgroup who elected to join this study of planned home births saw a doctor in labour. Ninety-three per cent of women in the planned home birth group were very satisfied with midwifery care, compared to 66% for doctor care where this was applicable. The comparable figures for the planned hospital delivery group were 90% and 67%, for here too the midwives were the prime carers. One way in which midwives compare well with doctors was described by this mother who had a home birth:

> The important thing (for me) is that I am listened to and not patronized, particularly by doctors who do not seem to have time to listen and always seem to be writing or opening mail or something else while consulting me. I find it very insulting. The midwives have always been pretty wonderful people.

According to one mother, the key role that midwives play in maternity care makes them the main hope for converting the rhetoric of *Changing Childbirth* into practice:

> If recent ideas in changes in childbirth are to work there will need to be major changes in attitudes towards all women wherever they choose to give birth. This will take a long time but I really feel that midwives should and must take the initiative. Midwives need to cut the rot that has set in and fall down hard on those in their midst who continue to pay little attention to freedom of choice and a woman's right to be in control.

Another mother, herself a midwife with the experience of conducting over 35 home deliveries, voiced the opinion of many when she immodestly claimed that:

> Midwives could carry the whole caseload of the UK, if rewarded and motivated, being confident in their skills to do so.

Paying for the maternity services

Many people were aware that what they want from the maternity services is increasingly constrained these days by the resources available:

My midwife was under tremendous pressure. The service she and her team offered was excellent but she was stressed. There are not enough midwives. The Government's so-called freedom of choice for women to choose the place where they give birth is a sham.

One mother expressed the hope that:

...there will not be cutbacks in the Health Service which lead midwifery to stop being a vocation and turn it into 'just a job' because then, women and midwives will miss out on an awfully important aspect of pregnancy and childbirth.

Many women commented on the generally negative impact of health service cuts on quality of care:

I feel that the care has been 'streamlined' in some ways. When I was expecting our first baby 8 years ago, my care was shared between the GP and midwife and I had the baby on the GP unit at the hospital and during the pregnancy antenatal classes were available. Two and a half years later when my second child was born, the GP unit no longer offered classes at their hospital due to lack of funding. Since having two more children at home, no advice was made available about breathing exercises except for what my midwife was able to offer during an antenatal visit which is time-limited.

Comparing experiences

Comparisons between different experiences of childbirth for women who have had more than one baby are useful, although the number of experiences must of necessity be small in each case. One mother who had had three babies summarized her experiences in the following terms:

What I most want from health care antenatally and postnatally:

(a) Personal care – care from as few professionals as possible;

(b) Group Midwifery – a group of midwives whom I can get to know who will provide continuity of care throughout pregnancy, labour and postnatally;

(c) Good postnatal support; and

(d) A breast-feeding counsellor.

In three pregnancies, I have received:

(1) *GP and consultant care* – no continuity of staff, very impersonal service. I was delivered by unknown midwife and hospital care was poor. The staff were too busy to give proper
support or care. Advice on breast-feeding and other items was
poor and inconsistent.

(2) *GP and midwifery care* – a planned home delivery which the
doctor refused to cover for. GP did all antenatal checks with
midwife in attendance – a waste of both their times and expertise. Little time to get to know midwife and discuss issues with
her. I was delivered by unknown midwife.

(3) *Midwifery care only* – antenatal care at home, plenty of time to
discuss things and get to know her. Group midwife setting. In
the last few weeks I knew when my midwife was on duty and
who was covering her off duty. Excellent continuity of care...

This process of reflecting on the quality of experiences in different birth
settings may also lead women to comment on the changes that have
occurred over time in maternity care. For some women, these have been
definitely beneficial:

Having had three children, all in hospital, I feel in the last 6 years
there has been a change in attitude towards maternity care in
hospitals and they have become friendlier and more comfortable
places to have your baby.

The management of childbirth varies not only over time but between
cultures. Thus, the issue of how birth is handled in other countries may
also come up. As another reasonably put it:

Both our children were born at home, one in the Netherlands, one
in the UK. Why is it so difficult to have home birth in this country?
... home birth should be given equally with the other options and
not presented as something foolhardy, only undertaken by cranks.

RECOMMENDATIONS FOR THE FUTURE

In reflecting on how birth had been for them, many of the people who
wrote comments on the follow-up questionnaire had suggestions to make
about how things might be improved in future. Their suggestions ranged

from extended paternity leave, to information leaflets about prenatal tests, to more frequent postnatal visits and better communication skills for health professionals.

One father was attracted by the sound of:

> ...the Dutch system, where home help comes to support parents, particularly mothers, after the birth – this is a sort of professional substitute for the old (now defunct) extended family. Also I would like to see paternity leave of 2 (or so) weeks to become legally entitled, as it seems unfair that men have to take holiday to be at home on anything but a holiday!

It was one mother's experience after a home birth that:

> ...it was quite hard waiting 24 hours for each midwife visit. For first-time mothers, the visits should be more frequent in the first two or three days while you get to grips with things. This would begin to compare with the on-call help other women receive in hospital.

– although not everyone who experienced hospital delivery would agree. Because of the need for more postnatal support, one mother decided that what she would really like would be a:

> ...reverse DOMINO – when you can go to hospital after a home birth to be looked after.

The isolation of many nuclear families today puts a greater premium on the role of fathers. One father's complaint about the timing of antenatal classes was echoed by several:

> NHS classes (antenatal) are run at 11 a.m. which almost seems a deliberate measure to exclude partners! If it wasn't for the NCT, I would have had to try and support my wife and communicate to the medical professionals without a clue as to what was happening! No wonder some fathers feel that they aren't involved. This must change. Run NHS classes in the evenings.

Simple measures could be taken to improve the quality of communication. One father thought it would be a good idea:

> To remind doctors and midwives not to look straight through husbands/partners when they ask questions and to introduce themselves to patients.

Men with a technological bent could see the advantages of extending to babies the care provided for computers:

> ...in this day and age families like ours are spread all over the country. Often the simple advice and day-to-day answers to our worries are not available or at least my wife feels 'silly' to ask and would rather worry than trouble the community staff at home. An advice line would be good! I have got one 24 hours [a day] with my computer!!!

CONCLUSIONS

The design of the Home Births Study cannot answer questions directly about the impact on women and their babies of different health settings, but can raise issues about differences and similarities[14]. The randomized controlled trial that is needed to provide definitive answers would be very difficult to organize, but has been shown to be feasible[15]. Were such a trial to be conducted, qualitative data collected from women would be likely to reinforce the main themes arising from other surveys, including this one by the National Birthday Trust Fund. Both the contrasts and the convergences are interesting. There is a contrast between accounts of hospital care that seems to remain impersonal, despite the improvements of recent years, and the warmth and support surrounding birth at home which lead most who have experienced it to regard it as a marvellous experience. There are also remarkably similar views expressed by most parents about what counts most in good maternity care: the quality of the relationship with the people providing it[16].

Much could be done to improve care both at home and in hospital without undertaking a randomized controlled trial to examine exactly what difference place of birth makes to women's experiences. Childbirth has a long way to go before the recommendations of *Changing Childbirth*[3] are likely to be seen in practice. For example, that report recommends that by 1998 75% of women should be delivered by a midwife they have got to know in pregnancy, and that:

> Women should receive clear, unbiased advice and be able to choose where they would like their baby to be born.

These conditions are far from being met at the present time. There is a clear need to continue to monitor women's experiences of maternity care, in order to have some measure of the extent to which, and direction in which, change is happening. The information arising from the National Birthday Trust Fund survey confirms the need for such monitoring of women's experiences to take account of the way in which recalled experiences, satisfaction and preferences may change over time[17-20].

The advantages that home birth may have to offer over hospital birth are likely to be a product of different factors. It may not be the setting itself, so much as the greater control and support from familiar people that seems to be possible at home. Such a conclusion emerges strongly from a recent Australian study[21]. No association was found between women's emotional well-being after birth and where the birth had happened, but factors such as a high obstetric procedure score, having unwanted people at the birth, experiencing poor postnatal care in hospital, not enough rest in hospital and being discharged too soon all made depression more likely. Other studies suggest that the quality of information and communication, which may also be better at home, is highly related to women's satisfaction[22].

The last word should be given to one of the women who took part in the follow-up survey. She had the opportunity of comparing birth at home with a previous birth in hospital. In her view, the two experiences were qualitatively different on several important dimensions. Both births were straightforward, but in hospital she was given different advice by different hospital staff and made to feel they were all too busy to answer her questions. This made her very depressed. By contrast:

> My home birth was absolutely wonderful. My care during pregnancy made me feel very special as the midwife and doctor both took extra interest. They would sit and listen to me without [the] distraction of a busy ward. We became friends and my family and I looked forward to the midwife's visits. She made me feel special and the birth was so special too ... I could go on for ages and ages about the wonderfulness of it all. I think my midwife deserves an award just for being great. She didn't do anything out of the ordinary, she just made me feel great.

ACKNOWLEDGEMENTS

I would like to thank Sandy Oliver for her invaluable comments, and Sandra Stone for help with wordprocessing.

REFERENCES

1. Cartwright, A. (1983). *Health Surveys in Practice and in Potential: A Critical Review of their Scope and Methods*. (London: King Edward's Hospital Fund)
2. Oakley, A. (1993). The follow-survey. In Chamberlain, G., Wraight, A. and Steer, P. (eds.) *Pain and its Relief in Childbirth*, pp. 101–13. (Edinburgh: Churchill Livingstone)
3. Department of Health (1993). *Changing Childbirth. Report of the Expert Maternity Group.* (London: HMSO)
4. Durward, L. and Evans, R. (1990). Pressure groups and maternity care. In Garcia, J., Kilpatrick, R. and Richards, A. (eds.) *The Politics of Maternity Care*, pp. 256–73. (Oxford: Clarendon Press)
5. Cartwright, A. (1979). *The Dignity of Labour?* (London: Tavistock)
6. Porter, M. and Macintyre, S. (1984). What is, must be best: a research note on conservative or deferential responses to antenatal care provision. *Soc. Sci. Med.*, **19**, 1197–1200
7. O'Brien, M. (1978). Home and hospital: a comparison of the experiences of mothers having home and hospital confinements. *J. Roy. Coll. Gen. Pract.*, **28**, 460–6
8. MacArthur, C., Lewis, M. and Knox, E.G. (1991). *Health after Childbirth.* (London: HMSO)
9. Kitzinger, S. (1978). Women's experiences of birth at home. In Kitzinger, S. and Davis, J.A. (eds.) *The Place of Birth.* (Oxford: Oxford University Press)
10. Kitzinger, S. (1979). *Birth at Home*, pp. 135–56. (Oxford: Oxford University Press)
11. O'Connor, M. (1995). *Birth Tides.* (London: Harper Collins)
12. Murphy-Black, T. (1994). Care in the community during the postnatal period. In Robinson, S. and Thomson, A.M. (eds.) *Midwives, Research and Childbirth*, Vol. 3, pp. 120–46. (London: Chapman Hall)
13. Mayall, B. and Foster, M.C. (1989). *Child Health Care: Living with Children, Working for Children.* (London: Heinemann)
14. Young, G. (1996). Uncertainty is likely to persist, but some knowledge would be better than none. *Br. Med. J.*, **312**, 755–6
15. Dowswell, T., Thornton, J.G., Hewison, J. and Lilford, R.J.L. (1996). Should there be a trial of home versus hospital delivery in the United Kingdom? *Br. Med. J.*, **213**, 753–5
16. Campbell, R. and Macfarlane, A. (1990). Recent debate on the place of birth. In Garcia, J., Kilpatrick, R. and Richards, A. (eds.) *The Politics of Maternity Care*, pp. 217–37. (Oxford: Clarendon Press)
17. Bennett, A. (1985). The birth of a first child: do women's reports change over time? *Birth*, **12**, 153–8
18. Jaccoby, A. and Cartwright, A. (1990). Finding out about the views and experiences of maternity-service users. In Garcia, J., Kilpatrick, R. and Richards, A. (eds.) *The Politics of Maternity Care.* (Oxford: Clarendon Press)
19. Oakley, A. (1980). *Women Confined: Towards a Sociology of Childbirth.* (Oxford: Martin Robertson)

20. Shaw, I. (1985). Reactions to transfer out of a hospital birth centre: a pilot study. *Birth,* **12**, 147–50

21. Brown, S., Lumley, J., Small, R. and Astbury, J. (1994). *Missing Voices: the Experience of Motherhood in Melbourne.* (Oxford: Oxford University Press)

22. Martin, C. (1990). How do you count maternal satisfaction? A user-commissioned survey of maternity services. In Roberts, H. (ed.) *Women's Health Counts*, pp. 147–66. (London: Routledge)

10

An economic evaluation of home births

Jane Henderson and Miranda Mugford

INTRODUCTION

This chapter compares the costs and benefits of home and hospital deliveries using data from the National Birthday Trust Fund (NBTF) survey. There has been some earlier work on the comparative costs of home and hospital deliveries[1,2]. Both found that total costs were lower for home births than hospital births, although not substantially so. They differed about whether or not the costs to the family were greater. This analysis provides a contemporary picture and considers costs affecting the National Health Service (NHS), the family and society.

METHODS

The intention at the outset was to compare the costs associated with births booked at 37 weeks gestation for home or hospital delivery, and to relate these costs to differences in outcome. Differences in cost alone would not be a sufficient reason for choice of place of delivery although it is an important consideration for the NHS. Clearly the decision also depends on the additional benefit to be gained. As there is no evidence that booked home delivery has an adverse effect on stillbirth or neonatal death rates[3], the decision must be based on other grounds including women's satisfaction. Costs were also estimated for unplanned home births but since the primary object of the survey was to examine planned births the data were very limited and costs could not be compared on the same basis. The approach we have followed is based on methods described by Drummond and co-workers[4].

We have based estimates of differences in health care activity and outcome on data from the NBTF survey. Questions were not asked directly about cost or financial consequences of home or hospital birth or about the numbers or place of antenatal visits. Where there were missing responses to questions, rates have been expressed using the number responding as the denominator. This assumes that the respondents were representative of the study population. Response rates to individual questions within the survey were higher than 93%.

The survey collected data about the use of health care at different stages in pregnancy, birth and in the postnatal period. We have done a retrospective costing of the available data. For each element of resource used, we estimated the cost of each unit of that resource. Unit cost data were available from various sources and are shown in the Appendix to this chapter. Estimates of each unit cost can vary depending on the sources; we have considered the effects of varying the costs between these limits in sensitivity analyses. These analyses systematically vary the values and assumptions employed in an evaluation in order to determine their implications for the results. The following aspects of the data were varied to test whether the results were sensitive to these factors.

(1)   The grade or scale of staff present (e.g. various grades of midwife; registrar or consultant obstetrician).

(2)   The time taken by staff to travel to and from the woman's home for booked home births.

(3)   The proportion of time staff were present in labour.

(4)   The costs of procedures including both materials and staff costs. Ninety-five per cent confidence limits were used for materials. For staff costs sensitivity limits were calculated by multiplying 95% confidence limits for time of procedure by the midpoint of the salary scale for staff present.

(5)   Increasing the duration of some procedures otherwise assumed to last for only 1 h. For example epidurals may be topped up every 2 h.

(6)   Some information was provided by both the women and the midwives (e.g. pain relief in labour). The effect of using one or other source was tested. Most of such information was taken from the midwife's questionnaire.

(7) For transfers; median travel times and distances were used in the main analysis and limits of inter-quartile ranges were used in the sensitivity analysis.

(8) Our assumptions about the composition of the transfer teams were also varied.

(9) Limits of inter-quartile ranges were used to test the effects of variation in length of postnatal stay.

(10) The expected lifetime of capital equipment carried by the community midwife and discount rates (which estimate today's valuation of future costs) applied. The number of home births attended per year were systematically varied.

All costs are shown at 1994 price levels, inflated or deflated where necessary by the Retail Price Index. Data were analysed using SPSS and Excel software packages.

RESULTS

Antenatal care

The survey was not concerned with antenatal visits so did not ask about the number or location of antenatal visits per woman. Types of antenatal care vary widely around the country[5,6] and women booked for home birth may have several hospital appointments for tests and scans. We have estimated costs to the NHS associated with antenatal visits at between £100 and £200 depending on the factors mentioned above.

Costs of antenatal tests reported are shown in Table 10.1. Overall, women booked for a hospital delivery were more likely to have a range of antenatal tests than those booked for home birth. Nearly all women had an ultrasound scan (95% of home booked, 99% of hospital booked). Data were not available on number of scans and it has been assumed that only one scan was performed. Nevertheless, at approximately £58 per scan this was a substantial cost component. The absolute cost may be an overestimate as it is based on data from the USA (see Appendix) but the estimate is the same for all groups and so is valid for comparisons. Other antenatal tests and procedures specifically mentioned included fetal cardiotocography (18% of home booked and 42% of hospital booked), amniocentesis (less than 5% of women) and Doppler (less than 3% of women) but these may be underestimates.

Table 10.1 Antenatal tests for women booked for home and hospital delivery: associated costs

Antenatal visits	Planned home births		Planned hospital births	
	% of women receiving tests	*Average cost cost per pregnancy* (£)	*% of women receiving tests*	*Average cost per pregnancy* (£)
Ultrasound scan	94.6	54.91	98.7	57.31
Cardiotocography	17.7	11.36	41.9	26.96
Amniocentesis	3.6	2.30	4.9	3.15
Doppler	2.3	0.89	1.7	0.65
Total		69.46		88.07
Mean no. responses	4630		3268	

Staff presence in labour and delivery

Table 10.2 shows the differences in staff present for women booked for home and hospital delivery and estimates of their associated costs. In this table women booked for home birth are subdivided by actual place of delivery. Eighty-three per cent of women booked and delivered at home had a G grade midwife attending compared to 46% of women booked for home birth but delivered in hospital, and 30% of women booked for a hospital delivery. Midwives graded E and F were more likely to attend women having a hospital delivery than home births. Medical staff were most likely to be present at deliveries booked for home birth but delivered in hospital compared with the other two groups.

Median durations of labour and delivery were longest in women booked for home birth but delivered in hospital (median duration of labour 465 min, delivery and third stage 27 min). Women booked and delivered at home had similar durations of labour and delivery to women booked for hospital birth (median length of labour at home was 306 min with median length of delivery and third stage 23 min compared with booked hospital labour of 290 min and a median length of delivery and third stage of 20 min).

For booked home births we have assumed that all staff also had a total of 30 min travelling time. The median travelling time for transfers, the majority of which were by car, was 15 min one way. With both hospital and home deliveries it is uncertain from questionnaire responses how much of the time the midwife was actually with the woman in labour,

Table 10.2 Staff present during labour and delivery at home and in hospital: associated costs (NBTF Home Births Survey 1994)

Staff	Home booked/ home delivered		Hospital booked/ hospital delivered		Home booked/ hospital delivered	
	% of women	Cost per woman (£)	% of women	Cost per woman (£)	% of women	Cost per woman (£)
Midwife						
E grade	1.5	0.60	30.1	9.97	15.7	6.35
F grade	6.0	2.75	14.8	5.87	9.6	4.48
G grade	82.8	43.46	29.9	17.05	45.6	24.32
H grade	2.6	1.52	1.3	0.76	2.1	1.24
I grade	0.4	0.26	0.2	0.13	0	0
Student midwife	14.0	4.88	21.4	66.92	18.5	6.31
General practitioner	11.4	3.25	2.5	0.42	8.1	1.57
Obstetrician	0.1	0.03	9.2	3.55	21.3	13.36
Anaesthetist	0	0	9.6	4.32	16.6	9.41
Paediatrician	0.2	0.14	13.0	2.84	11.3	11.10
Others	1.8	0.44	10.8	1.18	7.3	1.33
Total		60.15		47.27		81.28
No. responding	4182		3341		802	

particularly in the early stages. Our previous work on hospital deliveries has estimated that, on average, a midwife was present for about three-quarters of the duration of labour from the time of hospital admission[7]. We did not have information about the amount of time a midwife spent with women giving birth at home, but we have used this estimate of midwife presence in labour for both home and hospital deliveries. We have also assumed that other staff were present for 20% of the duration of labour and that all staff who were stated to be present at birth were there for the full duration of the second and third stages.

These data on staff presence, duration of labour and delivery, staff travel time for booked home births and percentage presence of staff were used to cost care for labour and delivery. The costs of staff varied from approximately £47 per woman for booked hospital births to £81 per woman for women booked for home birth but delivered in hospital. There was greater midwifery input to labours booked and delivered at home but more obstetric, anaesthetic and paediatric staff presence in hospital deliveries, particularly those that were booked for home birth.

Procedures, pain relief, mode of delivery and management of the third stage

Table 10.3 shows the variation in these aspects of care in labour for women booked and delivered at home, booked at home but delivered in hospital and booked hospital births. Induction, artificial rupture of the membranes, assisted and operative deliveries and all forms of medical pain relief were much less common in women booked and delivered at home. Women booked for home birth but delivered in hospital had higher rates of almost all interventions, particularly Caesarean section. Women booked for home births were more likely to use relaxation, massage and alternative therapies for pain relief. They were also more likely to have a physiologically managed third stage rather than one with an oxytocic drug and less likely to have any form of perineal trauma. The cost consequences of these variations are shown in Table 10.3. Overall, the reduced interventions associated with births booked and delivered at home resulted in costs £20 lower than booked hospital births which in turn were £20 lower than births booked for home but delivered in hospital.

Transfers

Six hundred women (15%) booked for a home birth were transferred to hospital during labour or immediately after. Of these, 91 were transferred after birth and 509 prior to birth. The other 179 women booked for home birth but delivered in hospital either changed their intention in the final weeks of pregnancy or the data relating to their transfer were incomplete. Table 10.4 shows the method of transfer and the associated costs. Almost half of the prenatal transfers were by car, a comparatively cheap form of transport. Most of the remaining prenatal transfers were by ambulance with a midwife, sometimes with a paramedic also in attendance. Postnatal transfers were on average more expensive and were most commonly by ambulance. The more costly obstetric and neonatal flying squads were used for only four transfers in this survey and a helicopter ambulance was needed on only one occasion. The final additional cost of transfers of women booked for home birth but delivered in hospital was estimated at £26.15 per woman transferred prior to delivery and £33.89 per woman transferred after delivery. Averaged over all women booked for home birth but admitted to hospital the cost of transfers was estimated at £27.33 per woman. The estimated extra cost averaged over all women booked for home birth was £3.29 per woman.

Table 10.3 Procedures, pain relief, mode of delivery and management of third stage : associated costs per woman. Data from midwives' returns (NBTF Home Births Survey 1994)

	Home booked/ home delivered		Hospital booked/ hospital delivered		Home booked/ hospital delivered	
	% of women	Cost per woman (£)	% of women	Cost per woman (£)	% of women	Cost per woman (£)
Procedures						
Induction	0.2	0.10	18.3	9.54	28.1	14.64
Artificial rupture of membranes	32.8	1.26	51.6	1.98	52.4	2.01
Mode of delivery						
Uncomplicated vaginal delivery (incl. breech)	100.0	11.01	90.5	9.96	72.7	8.00
Forceps	0	0	3.2	0.80	8.2	2.06
Ventouse	0	0	2.2	0.45	6.6	1.36
Caesarean section	0	0	4.2	3.50	12.5	10.41
Pain relief						
Entonox	50.3	0.56	72.1	0.81	66.0	0.74
Pethidine	4.3	0.05	30.3	0.33	23.1	0.25
Epidural	0	0	11.3	5.63	18.1	9.01
Spinal	0.1	0.05	1.3	0.65	4.1	2.04
General anaesthetic	0	0	2.2	1.26	4.4	2.52
Water birth	4.0	Not cost to NHS	1.0	0.23	0.2	0.04
Management of third stage						
Physiological	38.3	3.17	5.2	0.43	12.6	1.04
Manual removal of placenta	0.7	0.10	2.9	0.43	6.6	0.99
Syntometrine/ ergometrine	41.0	0.08	52.1	0.10	44.0	0.08
Syntocinon	0.9	0.01	7.2	0.06	11.6	0.10
Suturing perineum						
First-degree tear	23.7	1.57	19.7	1.30	12.4	0.82
Second-degree tear	20.8	2.12	23.8	2.43	19.8	2.02
Third-degree tear	0.1	0.04	0.4	0.11	0.3	0.08
Vaginal tear	5.8	0.69	0.5	0.06	6.4	0.77
Cervical tear	0	0.01	0.1	0.03	0.2	0.06
Episiotomy	2.4	0.29	13.1	1.57	20.6	2.47
Total		21.11		41.66		61.51
Mean no. responses	3502		3337		590	

Table 10.4 Method and cost of transfer of women booked for home birth (NBTF Home Births Survey 1994)

Method of transfer	Prenatal transfers		Postnatal transfers	
	% of women	Average cost per woman (£)	% of women	Average cost per woman (£)
Helicopter ambulance	0.02	1.76	0	0
Obstetric squad	0	0	2.2	1.20
Neonatal squad	0	0	1.1	0.74
Ambulance with paramedic	10.2	2.82	29.7	8.21
Ambulance with midwife	16.9	6.42	29.7	11.28
Ambulance with paramedic and midwife	16.1	6.12	25.3	9.61
Ambulance with GP	0.02	0.14	1.1	0.74
Ambulance	0.08	0.22	3.3	0.91
Car	55.6	8.67	7.7	1.20
Total	$n = 509$	26.15	$n = 91$	33.89

Care of baby

Table 10.5 shows care of the baby by intended and actual place of birth. Resuscitation was markedly more common among babies delivered in hospital with 21% of booked hospital births receiving resuscitation. Among babies booked for home birth but delivered in hospital 26% received resuscitation. Of babies booked and delivered at home 10.5% received resuscitation. This may be due to a lower threshold for resuscitation in hospital, the availability of equipment or skills and to differences in recording practice. The proportion of babies admitted to some form of neonatal special care was much higher in those booked for home births but delivered in hospital than in either of the other groups. There were insufficient data to cost this accurately, so it was assumed that average costs for Special Care Baby Units (SCBU) applied and that the babies were admitted for only a single day. This was the median length of stay for home born babies who were admitted. The length of stay of hospital born babies was not available. The cost consequences of these variations are shown in Table 10.5.

Equipment costs

Table 10.6 summarizes the data on equipment carried by the community midwives attending home births. Most midwives carried a mobile phone,

Table 10.5 Care of baby (NBTF Home Births Survey 1994)

Care of baby	Home booked/ home delivered		Hospital booked/ hospital delivered		Home booked/ hospital delivered	
	% of babies	*Cost per woman (£)*	*% of babies*	*Cost per woman (£)*	*% of babies*	*Cost per woman (£)*
Resuscitation	10.5	0.57	21.3	1.16	25.6	1.39
Special care baby unit	0.8	1.83	2.6	5.95	19.2	43.95
Total		2.40		7.11		45.34
No. in group	3896		3315		769	

a portable Doppler fetal heart monitor (Sonicaid), Entonox and equipment for neonatal resuscitation. The costs of these and other items are shown in Table 10.6. The most substantial costs were associated with the Entonox equipment and the Sonicaid but overall costs were estimated at less than £50 per home birth attended. Costs of capital equipment in the labour wards were estimated from the Women's Centre at the John Radcliffe Hospital, Oxford at £403 per week. With approximately 100 deliveries per week the cost per case was estimated at £4.

Daily hospital costs and total costs

Table 10.7 shows the estimated cost of a postnatal stay by intended and actual place of delivery. Women booked for hospital delivery had a median postnatal stay of 2 days (inter-quartile range 1–3 days). Our estimate of the marginal cost of an inpatient day was £72. It is important to distinguish this *marginal* cost from the *average* cost which includes the fixed costs of capital and overheads, and which is normally closer to the charges for hospital care which are often several hundreds of pounds per day. The marginal cost is that which changes with an additional unit of work-load. The resulting cost of £144 for a median of 2 days on the postnatal wards for hospital booked delivery represented over a quarter of the total antenatal, intrapartum and postnatal cost of a hospital birth. Women booked for a home birth but delivered in hospital had a median hospital stay of 1 day (inter-quartile range 1–2 days). The cost per woman in this group was estimated at £72. The cost averaged over all women booked for home birth was estimated at £13 per woman.

Table 10.6 Equipment carried by community midwife and associated costs (NBTF Home Births Survey 1994)

Equipment	% of midwives carrying equipment	Cost per home birth attended (£)*
Mobile phone	74.7	5.69
Radiopager	46.3	2.26
Sonicaid	77.2	12.14
Entonox	77.3	17.80
Oxygen for mother	42.0	1.51
Oxygen for baby	69.5	2.50
Bag/mask	75.1	6.95
Intravenous infusion set	42.6	0.03
Intravenous fluids	41.8	0.22
Neonatal narcan	53.9	0.46
Total		49.56

*Assuming that expected life of equipment was 5 years with a discount rate of 7%; that midwife attends four home births per year and that disposables were used or replaced four times per year

Table 10.7 summarizes the overall costs estimated for intrapartum and postnatal care. The estimated total average cost per woman home booked/home delivered was £205. For women booked for home birth but delivered in hospital the estimated cost was £405 and the estimated cost of a booked hospital birth was £332. The estimated total cost of a booked home birth irrespective of actual place of delivery was £237.

Costs to the family

These costs are summarized in Table 10.8. They do not include the travel cost of visits for antenatal care because these data were not collected in the survey. These costs were probably greater for women booked for hospital delivery since they were likely to have had more hospital visits. Women are frequently asked to pay themselves for the triple test for Down's syndrome but the proportions having this test were similar in the two groups, 3.3% of women booked for home delivery and 4.0% of women booked for hospital delivery. However, this was an open question and the figures are probably underestimates. Conversely women booked for home delivery may have paid to have an independent midwife or an alternative therapist such as an acupuncturist or a National Childbirth Trust teacher with them in labour. Three per cent hired a birth pool at a mean cost of £206.

Table 10.7 Daily hospital costs per woman (£) and summary of other costs to NHS

Summary of costs	Home booked/ home delivered	Home booked/ hospital delivered	All booked home	Hospital booked/ hospital delivered
Daily hospital costs*	1.80	71.99	13.12	143.98
Antenatal tests	69.52	69.52	69.52	88.17
Staff present in labour and delivery[†]	60.15	81.28	63.56	47.27
Procedures	1.36	16.65	3.83	11.52
Mode of delivery	11.01	21.83	12.75	14.71
Pain relief	0.66	14.60	2.91	8.91
Management of third stage	3.36	2.21	3.17	1.02
Suturing of perineum	4.72	6.22	4.96	5.50
Transfer	0.74	26.15	4.84	—
Care of baby	2.40	45.34	9.33	7.11
Equipment	49.56	49.56	49.56	4.03
Total	205.28	405.35	237.55	332.22
Total no. respondents	4191	806	4997	3470

* Based on median length of stay of home booked/hospital delivered of 1 day. Of those booked at home and delivered at home 2.5% were admitted postnatally. The median length of stay of hospital booked/hospital delivered was 2 days
[†]Including travel costs where appropriate

It is also probable that the women's partner would have taken more time off work if she had a home birth. We have made a conservative estimate of 2 additional days. The social class distribution of women intending home and hospital births and their partners are shown in Table 10.9.

Women booked for home delivery and their partners had higher status occupations than those intending hospital delivery. This may affect the family's costs in a number of ways. Paternity leave is probably more commonly available to those in professional and managerial occupations. Similarly, annual leave entitlements are generally more generous for people in non-manual occupations. Thus it is possible that men in manual occupations may be worse off financially if their partner opts for a home birth since they may be obliged to take unpaid leave. Overall it is difficult to judge the effect on family costs but our estimates are dominated by partners' lost production. Even if this factor is excluded, having the birth at home cost the family nearly three times as much as having it in hospital.

Table 10.8 Costs to the family (NBTF Home Births Survey 1994)

	Booked home birth		Booked hospital birth	
		Cost (£)		Cost (£)
Triple test	3.3%	2.12	4.0%	2.57
Independent midwife	4.7%	2.83	0.1%	1.81
Acupuncturist*	0.5%	0.50	—	—
National Childbirth Trust teacher*	0.1%	0.10	—	—
Hire of birth pool	3.4%	7.00	—	—
Partner's time lost from paid work†	x plus 2 days	300.00	x days	—
Total		312.55		4.38
No. responding	4997		3506	

*Assuming present for 4 hours at £25 per hour
†Assuming that partner takes an extra 2 days off work at £150 per day (these data were not collected in the survey)

Costs in other parts of the economy

Costs to society through lost production may be greater following home births if partners take more time off work. If the company arranges additional staff cover for them this would incur costs to the company. If the partners of women in either group take unpaid leave, there will be a reduction in tax revenue which is a cost to the Treasury. The losses and gains arising from paternity or annual leave cannot easily be predicted, however. For example, self-employed men may lose more through taking time off than men employed by an organization. Men employed on piece rates may also lose more. Overall, if there is any loss of production from partners' paternity leave, it is likely to be higher for the home birth group.

The marked differences in method of infant feeding (Table 6.10, Chapter 6) may also incur differences in costs to the NHS and society. Among women booked for home birth, 80% were exclusively breast-feeding their babies 2 days postnatally compared with only 58% of those booked for hospital delivery. At 6–8 weeks 66% of women booked for home birth and 44% of women booked for hospital birth were still exclusively breast-feeding. In addition, a higher proportion of those intending to breast-feed succeeded in doing so – 94% of women booked for home birth compared to 88% of women booked for hospital birth.

The ramifications of these differences in the long term are difficult to quantify. It has been suggested that babies who were breast-fed are less likely to require health care in early childhood[8,9]. Breast-feeding mothers

Table 10.9 Social class distribution of women and their partners by intended place of birth (NBTF Home Births Survey 1994)

Social class	Women		Partners of women	
	Booked home deliveries (%)	Booked hospital deliveries (%)	Booked home deliveries %	Booked hospital deliveries (%)
I	4.6	2.9	10.3	8.0
II	34.6	21.6	32.3	24.1
IIIn	26.4	39.3	14.0	15.6
IIIm	9.0	10.1	26.7	33.4
IV	3.9	7.2	7.0	10.6
V	0.5	0.8	1.4	2.5
Student	0	0	0	3.6
Housewife	20.8	18.0	4.6	0.9
Armed forces	0.2	0.1	2.1	1.3
Total responses	4997	3470	4974	3470

may also require less health care and therefore should not be prevented from returning to work because of morbidity than bottle-feeding mothers. However, it is equally possible that women breast-feeding may have more problems returning to work[10]. If women return to work earlier following a home birth, this would lead to lower net social costs than booking for hospital birth.

Unplanned home births

The survey was commissioned to examine planned home and hospital births and the data collected on unplanned home births were minimal. Therefore they cannot be compared with the booked births. A brief estimate of their associated costs to the NHS for intrapartum care is shown in Table 10.10.

These women were relatively unsupported in labour and birth. Nearly half were delivered by a midwife and a third had an ambulance officer present. Forty-one per cent were transferred to hospital, generally by ambulance, and 19% of babies were admitted to SCBU. If one assumes that these women stayed only 1 day in hospital, the cost to the NHS per woman was estimated at about £100 but this does not include antenatal care and may grossly underestimate the true costs.

Table 10.10 Unplanned home births (NBTF Home Births Survey 1994)

	% of women	*Average cost per woman (£)*
*Staff present**		
Ambulance officer	29.2	3.27
Midwife	48.4	5.72
General practitioner	7.4	2.19
Obstetrician	0.5	0.15
Others	3.2	0.25
		subtotal = 11.58
Transfers		
Helicopter	0.1	0.87
Obstetric squad	1.3	0.53
Neonatal squad	0.6	0.25
Ambulance with paramedic	16.4	4.53
Ambulance with midwife	12.8	4.20
Ambulance with both	9.4	3.09
Car	0.8	0.04
Total requiring transfer	41.5	subtotal = 13.51
Procedures		
Manual removal of placenta	1.3	0.19
Blood transfusion	0.5	0.16
Repair of tear (second degree)	16.2	1.65
Delivery of placenta	2.9	0.03
Baby admitted to SCBU	18.9	43.26
		subtotal = 45.29
Daily hospital cost	41.3	29.73
Total cost to NHS		100.11
No. responses	1587	

*Assuming that staff present for 1 h

Sensitivity analysis

Extreme scenarios were used to estimate the highest and lowest likely costs for booked home and hospital deliveries. Costs for antenatal visits and tests, staff presence in labour and delivery, procedures and pain relief in labour, perineal damage, and most importantly, days in hospital, all confirmed the greater cost of hospital delivery. This cost was consistently exceeded by the small group of women who were booked for home birth but were transferred for delivery in hospital.

Management of the third stage was more often without oxytocic drugs (physiological) in home delivered babies. This was more costly because of the greater staff time involved assuming that such a physiologically managed third stage may last up to 1 h. Admission to some form of SCBU was much more frequent in babies booked for home birth but delivered in hospital and the cost of this may be considerable. The overall cost of transfer to hospital was low, due to the relatively low percentage needing transfer and the relatively low cost of the predominant form of transfer, by car.

Equipment carried by the community midwife was valued at approximately £50 per home birth attended. We varied the expected lifetime of equipment between 3 and 7 years, discount rates between 5% and 10% and the number of home births attended between two and six per year. This produced an upper limit of £165 which would make it almost as costly as a booked hospital delivery, and a lower limit of £23. If the equipment was used more efficiently, for example, if a midwife attended more home births or if the equipment was shared between a group, these costs would be much less. If the same equipment was used for 20 home births the cost would be about £10 per home birth attended.

Using average or median costs and durations, as in the main analysis, the difference between the total costs of the two groups by booking intention was just under £100 per woman. If low costs and short durations of procedures and lengths of stay were assumed throughout, booked hospital delivery was still more expensive by nearly £50 per woman. If high costs and long durations were assumed, hospital deliveries were more costly by over £300 per woman. Women booked for home birth but delivered in hospital were the most cost intensive group. The analysis was sensitive to the assumptions made about staff input, which was higher in this group, and the level of care and length of stay in neonatal intensive care, which was also highest in this group. Using the costings from the main analysis, approximately two-thirds of women booked for home birth would have had to be admitted to hospital for their costs to equate to those of booked hospital births. Since only 16% of women booked for home birth were actually admitted, this resulted in substantially lower costs.

DISCUSSION

These analyses were by the place of birth intended at 37 weeks with booked home births subdivided by actual place of delivery. There were striking variations in many aspects of care including rates of Caesarean sections, epidural anaesthetics and episiotomies. However, this was not a randomized trial and some selection biases are inevitable. Women who choose to have a home birth are not representative of the general population. They are a self-selected group who are, on average, better educated, of higher social class and are probably used to having more power of decision-making. The controls in this survey were selected by midwives on the basis of their general similarity (in age group, parity and obstetric background). It is thus not possible to say with certainty that the generally better outcomes for women who had home births, (in terms of satisfaction with care, breast-feeding rates, intact perineum – see Chapters 6 and 7) were due to place of birth. These results could also be due to these women being committed to a non-interventionist approach, representing the Natural Childbirth lobby in greater proportion than women booked for hospital delivery. It is important to remember that if the popularity of home birth continues to increase, then they will become more representative of the general population and those apparent benefits of home birth which are in fact due to selection will be reduced.

There may also be response bias. The overall response rate to joining the survey was relatively low (61%) of all births at home in the UK in 1994 (98% of those who registered in the study) but of those who did join, response rates did not show any disinclination of reporting among those who had a bad experience of home birth. A sample follow-up of non-responders found, reassuringly, that their outcome was not significantly different but that they had a slightly higher induction rate. This would have the effect of narrowing the cost difference between the two groups. Because of these possibilities for serious bias, we have considered it inappropriate to calculate cost-effectiveness ratios for any outcomes.

The only group that had significantly higher stillbirth and neonatal death rates was that of women with unplanned home births. Limited data on this group of women suggest much lower levels of support in labour and higher transfer rates with low overall costs. However, data were not available on many aspects of their care so this low costing figure is incomplete. Moreover, unplanned home birth would never be a policy option.

The unit costs shown in the Appendix to this chapter were a mixture of average costs and marginal costs and came from a variety of sources. Marginal costs exclude the fixed cost element such as capital and overheads and are thus considerably less than hospital charges. In a short-term analysis such as this it would have been preferable to use marginal costs throughout but these were not always available. Much of the unit cost data on procedures, pain relief and mode of delivery were collected as part of a European study of care during labour[7,11] and refer to the marginal costs of staff and materials for procedures averaged over six centres in the UK. Where other unit cost data were not available, average extra contractual referral tariffs in the Oxford and Anglia Region were used. These were probably somewhat higher than the true average costs but when they were varied in the sensitivity analysis, it made little difference.

Staff costs were based on the pay scales in place in 1994, increased by 20% to allow for employment costs such as superannuation and training. If home birth continues to become more popular, the training of additional midwives to work independent of the consultant unit and the supply of the necessary support (equipment, back-up staff, emergency cover) will become a real, rather than simply a theoretical cost.

CONCLUSIONS

Although we have estimated a lower average cost of home birth based on current practice, extra resources will be required in the short term if home births continue to increase in popularity. This is because the shift to the community would not immediately free resources in the hospital maternity unit except by allowing staff more time to spend with women. All hospital services would still need to remain available. The shift to the community would have to be very large before cost savings could be seen in the release of hospital staff or space.

The better outcome alongside the lower expected costs per case lead us to conclude that the recommendations in *Changing Childbirth*[12] of a real option of a home birth for all women who want it would also be a cost-effective option.

ACKNOWLEDGEMENTS

Our grateful thanks to the staff of the National Perinatal Epidemiology Unit and the editors for their helpful comments. The authors are funded by the Department of Health.

Appendix to Chapter 10

Unit costs of various items and procedures, 1994 price levels: costs include both staff and materials

	Unit costs	95% Confidence limits or range of values*		Reference
		Low	High	
Antenatal care				
Outpatient appointment	64.35	53.03	75.67	13–17
Ultrasound scan	58.06	16.97	99.15	18
Alpha fetoprotein	2.88	—	—	Shackley*
Amniocentesis	312.73	—	—	Twaddle*
Doppler	19.86	22.54	38.38	18
Fetal cardiotocography	20.72	9.82	27.92	18
Triple test	64.35	53.03	75.67	18
Pain relief				
Entonox	1.12	0.53	1.69	7
Pethidine	1.10	0.59	2.08	11
Epidural/spinal	49.79	35.50	83.21	11
General anaesthetic	57.28	32.51	83.96	11
Water birth – (hospital)	22.52	5.14	87.32	†
(hired for home)	206.00	178.22	234.09	†
Procedures				
Induction	52.11	41.97*	62.24*	19
Artificial rupture of membranes	3.84	3.27	5.39	11
Mode of delivery				
Uncomplicated vaginal delivery	11.01	5.83	24.11	11
Forceps	25.13	15.19	51.43	11
Ventouse	20.57	10.01	43.79	11
Caesarean section	83.25	51.76	155.86	11
Third stage				
Physiological	8.27	2.01	30.32	11
Manual removal of placenta	14.98	7.20	33.36	11
Syntometrin/ergometrine	0.19	—	—	7
Syntocinon	0.89	—	—	7

Method of transfer[‡]	Journey time			Reference
	30 min	*20 min*	*40 min*	
Obstetric squad	41.00	21.83	95.49	18, 20, 21
Neonatal squad	41.00	21.83	95.49	18, 20, 21
Ambulance with paramedic	27.65	14.39	43.18	18, 20, 21
Ambulance with midwife	32.82	17.56	50.76	18, 20, 21
Ambulance with paramedic and midwife	32.82	17.56	50.76	18, 20, 21
Car (35p per mile)	5.18	3.17	7.58	18, 20, 21
Helicopter	867.39	395.76	1640.59	22
Ambulance	27.65	14.39	43.18	18, 20, 21
Ambulance with general practitioner	47.63	26.35	73.12	18, 20, 21

	Unit costs	95% Confidence limits		Reference
		Low	*High*	
Baby care				
Resuscitation	5.43	1.94	12.91	11
SCBU	228.89	145.66	572.22	23
Repair of episiotomy or tear				
First-degree tear	6.61	2.74	21.58	11
Second-degree tear	10.19	7.16	18.02	11
Third-degree tear	28.29	11.83	48.72	11
Vaginal tear	11.97	7.05	24.04	11
Cervical tear	28.29	11.83	48.72	11
Episiotomy	11.97	7.05	24.04	11
Equipment carried by midwife				
Mobile phone	125.00	—	—	J. Knowles*
Radiopager	80.00	—	—	J. Knowles*
Sonicaid	258.00	—	—	J. Knowles*
Entonox	377.76	—	—	J. Knowles*
Intravenous infusion set	1.06	—	—	J. Knowles*
Intravenous fluids	8.56	—	—	J. Knowles*
Neonatal narcan	13.92	—	—	J. Knowles*
Laerdal bag/mask	135.00	—	—	J. Knowles*
Oxygen	117.76	—	—	J. Knowles*
Daily hospital costs	71.99	14.88	129.10	7

Staff costs (rate/h)	Midpoint	Lowpoint	Highpoint	Reference
Midwives				
Grade D	7.85	7.33	8.41	20, 21
Grade E	8.98	8.41	9.73	20, 21
Grade F	10.35	9.32	11.41	20, 21
Grade G	11.84	10.98	12.71	20, 21
Grade H	13.15	12.27	14.03	20, 21
Grade I	14.48	13.59	15.40	20, 21
Senior house officer	12.55	11.06	14.03	20, 21
Registrar	13.81	12.54	15.21	20, 21
Senior registrar	16.36	14.44	18.28	20, 21
Consultant	29.61	25.84	33.37	20, 21
Ambulance officer	11.20	10.71	13.39	20, 21
Acupuncturist	25.00	24.00	30.00	§
Aromatherapist	25.50	25.00	28.00	§

*Personal communication
†Data collected in survey for project on water births NPEU Oxford, 1995
‡Confidence limits are low and high points on the pay scales for various staff applied to the median and quartile values for journey time
§Sample of practices in Oxford

REFERENCES

1. Ferster, G. and Pethybridge, R.J. (1973). The costs of a local maternity care system. *Hosp. Health Service Rev.*, July, 243–7
2. Stilwell, J.A. (1979). Relative costs of home and hospital confinement. *Br. Med. J.*, **2**, 257–9
3. Campbell, R. and Macfarlane, A. (1994). *Where to be Born?* (Oxford: National Perinatal Epidemiology Unit)
4. Drummond, M.F., Stoddart, G.L. and Torrance, G.W. (1987). *Methods for the Economic Evaluation of Health Care Programmes*. (Oxford: Oxford Medical Publications)
5. Sikorski, J., Wilson, J., Clement, S., Das, S. and Smeeton, N. (1996). A randomized controlled trial comparing two schedules of antenatal visits: the antenatal care project. *Br. Med. J.*, **312**, 546–5
6. Tucker, J.S., Hall, M.H., Howie, P.W., Reid, M.E., Barbour, R.S., Florey, C. du V. and McIlwaine, G.M. (1996). Should obstetricians see women with normal pregnancies? A multicentre randomised controlled trial of routine antenatal care by general practitioners and midwives compared with shared care led by obstetricians. *Br. Med. J.*, **312**, 554–9
7. Mugford, M. (1996). *How does the method of cost estimation affect the assessment of cost-effectiveness in health care*. DPhil Thesis University of Oxford, Oxford
8. Howie, P.W., Forsyth, S., Ogston, S.A., Clark, A. and Florey, C. du V. (1990). Protective effect of breast feeding against infection. *Br. Med. J.*, **300**, 11–16

9. Standing Committee on Nutrition of the British Paediatric Association. (1994). Is breast feeding beneficial in the UK? *Arch. Dis. Child.*, **71**, 376–80

10. Brown, S., Lumley, J., Small, R. and Astbury J. (1994). *Missing Voices: Experience of Motherhood.* (Melbourne: Oxford University Press)

11. Mugford, M. (1993). The cost of continuous electronic fetal monitoring in low risk labour. In Spencer, J.A.D. and Ward, R.H.T. (eds.) *Intrapartum Fetal Surveillance.* (London: RCOG Press)

12. Department of Health. (1993). *Changing Childbirth.* (London: HMSO)

13. DeVore, G.R. (1994). The routine antenatal diagnostic imaging with ultrasound study: another perspective. *Obstet. Gynecol.*, **84**, 622–6

14. Temmerman, M. and Buckene, P. (1991). Cost effectiveness of routine ultrasound in first trimester pregnancies. *Europ. J. Obstet. Gynecol. Reprod. Biol.*, **39**, 3–6

15. Hahn, R., Ho, S., Roi, H., Bulgarin-Viera, M., Davies, T. and Macmillan, W. (1988). Cost effectiveness of office obstetrical ultrasound in family practice: preliminary considerations. *J. Am. Board Fam. Pract.*, **1**, 33–8

16. Hillman, B., Joseph, C., Marby, M., Sunshine, J., Kennedy, S. and Noether, M. (1990). Frequency and cost of diagnostic imaging in office practice – a comparison of self-referring and radiologist-referring physicians. *N. Engl. J. Med.*, **323**, 1604–8

17. Pitkin, R. (1991). Screening and detection of congenital malformations. *Am J. Obstet. Gynecol.*, **164**, 1045–8

18. Anglia and Oxford Regional Health Authority. (1995). Extra contractual referral tariffs 1994–95. NHS Executive

19. Davies, L. and Drummond, M. (1993). The costs of induction of labour by prostaglandin E_2 or oxytocin: refining the estimates. Discussion paper 109. (York: Centre for Health Economics)

20. Review body on doctors' and dentists' remuneration. (1994) *Twenty-third report.* (London: HMSO)

21. Review body for nursing staff, midwives, health visitors and professions allied to medicine. (1994). *Eleventh Report on Professions Allied to Medicine.* (London: HMSO)

22. Snooks, H., Nicholl, J., Brazier, J. and Lees-Mlanga, S. (1996). Costs and benefits of helicopter emergency ambulance services in England and Wales. *J. Publ. Health Med.*, **18**, 67–77

23. Mugford, M. (1994). Outcome and cost of neonatal intensive care. *Curr. Paediatr.*, **4**, 30–2

11

Implications of the findings of the survey

This survey is semi-quantitative and many implications have been derived from the open questions. The authors of the report present some of the implications of the results for consideration. This is presented in four groups, the women seeking home births, the midwives who are the major providers of home care, the doctors including general practitioners (GPs) who may be involved in home births or hospital delivery, and the health authorities who have to plan for any changes in the future of home births and find funds for these schemes.

IMPLICATIONS FOR WOMEN

The findings of this study are of considerable interest to women who are either currently pregnant or intending to have babies in the future. We may hope that this study will inform them about the safety of home birth and the degree of satisfaction experienced by women delivering both at home and in hospital (Chapter 7). As this was not a randomized trial, the study findings must be interpreted in the light of a selection bias at entry from those women who were willing to take part and an ascertainment bias after delivery; women or midwives from either arm of the study may have been less likely to complete questionnaires after delivery in cases where the outcome was poor. To reduce these biases, a follow-up of non-responders has resulted in us obtaining minimal outcome data for all but 1% of those registered in the survey who were intending home birth and 2% of those intending hospital birth (Chapter 3).

Information

The study findings suggest that most women who deliver in hospital have made that decision before pregnancy or soon after becoming pregnant while women who plan a home birth decide later (Chapter 7). We were not convinced that either group had access to good quality information about all options available, in the spectrum from a consultant bed in a hospital, through GP units, DOMINO schemes to home deliveries with community or independent midwives. The risks of home birth may have been exaggerated by some doctors while the harsh picture of hospital birth drawn by some anti-hospital protagonists does not match that described by many of the study participants (Chapter 7). Even the information leaflets provided by the Midwives' Information and Resource Service (MIDIRS) and the Royal College of Obstetricians and Gynaecologists (RCOG) may still contain information that is unwittingly partial[1].

These biases make it difficult for women who are attempting to make an informed choice and may even be hazardous. A biased view about the place of birth may cause a woman unsuitable for home birth to persist in her plan, her resolve having been hardened by opposition to her plans for home delivery. The dearth of good quality unbiased information for women should be rectified preferably by written guidelines in each health authority including local variation of what is really available in the domiciliary or hospital setting. Perhaps an independent group of professional (e.g. public health doctors) could edit such advisory material which has been prepared by unwittingly biased obstetricians or midwives.

Women considering home birth should be aware that many modern GPs have little experience of domiciliary birth and that the training they have received as house officers in obstetrics and gynaecology often left them knowing a great deal less about normal labour and delivery than experienced midwives. In the past, GPs could assist at home birth by performing a forceps delivery for delay in the second stage of labour or fetal distress. However, by 1994 not a single such delivery by a GP was recorded in this study. The reality is that despite their statutory requirement to assist if called to give medical aid at a home birth, the majority of modern GPs seem unwilling to assist at simple vaginal operative deliveries and have less to offer in this aspect than previous generations of family doctors.

Satisfaction

Women who wish to deliver at home are very different from those intending a hospital birth. Lack of interference in labour, freedom of choice, the convenience of being at home, were priorities for these women both in deciding to deliver at home and in rating satisfaction with the experience afterwards (Chapter 7). Safety was not mentioned by these women as a reason for choosing home birth and fear of an adverse outcome rated as a drawback to home birth by only 6%.

Women choosing to deliver in hospital are strongly motivated by safety for themselves and their babies when deciding where to deliver and in rating satisfaction afterwards. The most important implication of the study for women is that despite the fundamental differences in outlook of the two groups of women and their very different experiences at the time of birth, 98% of women in both groups were either satisfied or very satisfied with their care. The decision on where to deliver does not affect satisfaction; however, the success in achieving home delivery has a major effect. Those who wished to deliver at home and succeeded in so doing were the most satisfied while those who delivered in hospital following transfer from home were, not surprisingly, the least (Chapters 4, 7 and 9).

It came as no surprise to find that women who planned to deliver at home and did so, liked being in their own homes, feeling stress-free, in control and close to their families. Women considering home birth might be interested in some of the negative aspects of home birth that these women encountered. The continued burdens of housework, interruptions by visitors and families and the mess associated with home birth were commented upon. Women who delivered in hospital liked feeling safe, getting lots of help and enjoyed the company of other women and the freedom from housework. Unsatisfactory aspects of hospital care tended to relate more to the postnatal period and facilities rather than to delivery; in the hospital environment there were unacceptable rules, routines and procedures which were distasteful to many women. Noise, lack of good bathing and lavatory facilities and the quality of the food were other sources of discomfort for many women (Chapter 7).

Midwives, doctors and women have conducted or participated in many clinical trials aimed at finding effective and satisfactory care for women in pregnancy and childbirth[2]. Some forms of care have been shown to be either of no value or to be less effective than alternatives. Consumers will be disappointed to note that among both arms of the study women received forms of care that have been demonstrated to be ineffective or harmful. Only 16% of those who delivered at home as planned and 26% of those who delivered in hospital as planned had perineal injuries sutured with man-made absorbable materials (vicryl or dexon), despite good quality evidence that their use is associated with less pain and dyspareunia than catgut (Chapter 5). Half of the women delivering in hospital were not allowed to drink during labour despite the lack of evidence to support this restriction (Chapter 4).

Women delivering at home were more likely to have met their midwife beforehand and while this was rated as important by 8% of women, it had little effect on the progress or safety of the labour (Chapter 7). The attendance at a home birth by a known midwife is an aspiration that cannot always be met. It may be purchased at some cost by women who chose to be attended by an independent midwife, but even independent midwives have personal lives and domestic commitments that make constant availability sometimes unrealistic. Some of the women participating in this study were unrealistic in their demands for the constant availability and continued care throughout labour of a named midwife regardless of the duration of labour, duty rosters, lack of overtime pay and the midwife's family commitments (Chapter 7). The study revealed a very high level of satisfaction expressed by women with midwifery care at home and in hospital even from midwives they had never met before labour. Realistic expectations about continuity of care must be explained beforehand so as to prevent the birth being spoiled by disappointment at the presence of a hitherto unknown midwife.

Safety

We were aware from the outset that neither the design nor the size of this study would allow confident statements to be made about the maternal or perinatal safety of home or hospital births. The overall perinatal outcome in the study appears to be excellent, although we cannot exclude the possibility of an excess of adverse outcomes among those who would not join the study (Chapter 3) and the unbooked home deliveries (Chapter 8).

In this study among the low-risk women intending home birth there was at least a 16% chance of transfer to hospital, increasing to 40% among women having their first babies. Multigravidae who had a Caesarean section in a previous delivery had a 28% admission rate to hospital for delivery, over twice that of the multiparae booking for home birth (Chapter 4). Transfer to hospital was often an upsetting event that adversely affected a woman's satisfaction with her care. Typically it took up to 15 min to summon help to the home and up to half an hour to get to hospital. The pain, risk and stress associated with this journey varied with the indication for transfer and the distance between home and hospital. A long journey with minimal analgesia during a delayed second stage of labour is obviously much more distressing than transfer before labour for assessment of prolonged pregnancy.

Intended home birth is associated with a lower risk of instrumental delivery and delivery by Caesarean section overall. The lower maternal intervention rates may be a real benefit of home birth or may result from the biases already mentioned. Among those transferred from home to hospital, however, the rates for all maternal and neonatal interventions increased greatly.

Conclusions

Good quality information about local facilities and all options for delivery available to women should be laid out. Information about the general and specific risks of home and hospital birth should be communicated to women in an objective manner. Distance from hospital, potential speed and convenience of transfer in an emergency need to be considered. Women having their first babies should give careful consideration to the high likelihood of transfer during labour with all its attendant distress as should multiparae who had a previous Caesarean section. Early discharge from hospital to home or to GP units should be facilitated for those women who actually request it and every effort should be made to improve the toilet facilities, food and midwifery care in postnatal wards.

IMPLICATIONS FOR MIDWIVES

The number of births in the UK taking place in the home decreased from 35% in the 1960s to 1% in the 1980s rising slightly to 1.9% in the mid-1990s (Chapter 1). Midwives who qualified when the home birth rate was as high as 35% would be nearing the end of their careers when this study was conducted in 1994 and this group would probably represent a small percentage of the midwives who took part. Many midwives would have trained in the 1980s when the home birth rate was at its lowest, allowing little opportunity to provide intranatal care in the home. Does the lack of experience in home births have any bearing on the midwife's skills, her ability to adapt to a different environment and to provide the necessary care to mother and baby?

Cronk[3] argues that:

> If midwives are to become confident about home births, they need time to study and adapt to the responsibilities associated with it.

Training

In this study, the midwives were asked if they had received any theoretical or practical training relating to home birth in the past 2 years. Less than a third (31%) reported that they had had some theory and less than half (44%) had practical training. Many, who had had no training, qualified their answers by writing comments on this issue and they seemed quite indignant that the question suggested that training specific to home birth was needed.

> I feel strongly that a midwife's training and clinical competence should enable her to adapt confidently and competently to any surroundings.

> What do you need? I can deliver a baby. What else is there?

These comments put to one side the need for a team approach particularly in the face of problems. Some midwives felt that practical training is difficult to provide since there are few people experienced enough in home births to feel qualified to teach others.

> Who would give me this 'training'? – people who have far less experience than myself!

Midwives, who work permanently in the community spend some time, often 1 week a year, on the labour ward to update their skills in intranatal care. Perhaps some midwives did not relate this training to home births, although some did:

> Study days and lunch time sessions may be relevant to some aspects of home births and are available, i.e. management of labour, resuscitation of the newborn.

Midwives need to be aware of current research so that they can update their practice as necessary according to the findings and evidence produced by that particular piece of work. One example is the availability of new materials for perineal repair known to absorb more completely and cause less discomfort during the healing process. In this study, it was disappointing to learn that two-thirds of perineal repairs in the home birth group were done using catgut. In this group, three-quarters of the repairs were performed by midwives.

Very few midwives expressed anxiety about their lack of knowledge or expertise in home births, or the need for additional training. One midwife, however, commented:

> The last time I delivered a baby at home was 18 years ago. I am a little concerned that younger midwives are being encouraged to undertake home deliveries with no practical training.

In the recent Department of Health report *Changing Childbirth*[4], the emphasis was on women-centred and community-based care. Although it was agreed that student midwives should be competent to practise in both community and hospital settings before registration, the report also stated that:

> Midwives who have been in practice for some time without undertaking their full role may need support for professional development and in the updating of some of their skills (p. 39).

These are soft words but their meaning is clear: to look after home deliveries needs skills which not all younger midwives have honed. Perhaps as worrying are the midwives who have not been in practice for some time (Chapter 7).

One husband, whose wife gave birth in hospital as planned, wrote the following comment:

> The main reason for not having a home birth was the risk attached. If the Health Service was more flexible and allowed professionals with the correct experience and equipment to help with all home births, then the risk could be lessened and people's confidence raised. At present you are likely to get doctors and even midwives who are inexperienced with, and often opposed to, home births. Unless you are sure of confident technicians you are unlikely to be confident yourself.

Experience of home births

The midwives were asked about the number of home births at which they had assisted in the past year. Figure 11.1 shows the results.

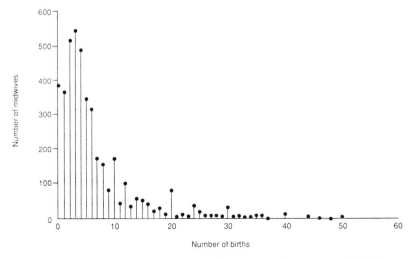

Figure 11.1 Number of home births attended by midwives in past year (NBTF Home Births Survey 1994)

In this study 2811 midwives (64%) had attended five or fewer home births (see Table 11.1) and 383 of this group had no previous experience at all inside a year.

An examination of the regional breakdown of these same data (Table 11.1 and Figure 11.2) showed the great variety of past experience midwives had of home births in the last year. Over half of the midwives in South East Thames and South Western Regions had delivered 6–20 women but in several regions, over 80% of midwives had attended fewer than six births. Northern Ireland led in the inexperience rate but only 23 home births were reported there in the year. Perhaps more serious were the Northern Region (96% of 110 births), Scotland (90% of 197) and the West Midlands, the largest of the old regions with 84% of 323 home births attended by midwives who had delivered five or fewer women at home in the previous year. Such regional fluctuations are based on small numbers but still reflect a worrying picture in some areas of the country.

In a small study conducted by Floyd in 1992[5], a similar situation was reported. Thirty-two per cent of the midwives who participated had no experience of home birth in the previous year and 46% had witnessed or conducted only one or two births in the home.

In this National Birthday Trust Fund (NBTF) study, few midwives (4%) had attended more than 20 home births in the past year. Sixty-one per cent of this group nationally were independent midwives. Community midwives' groups, dedicated to provide care to women who have chosen

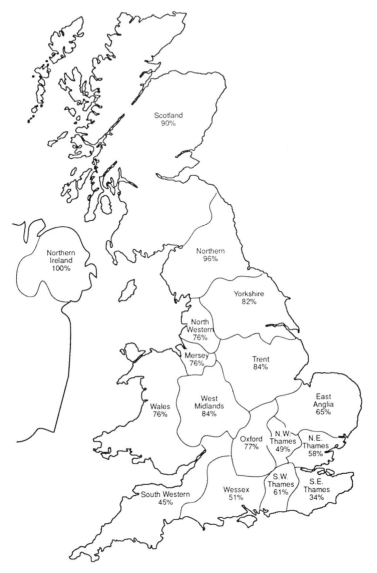

Figure 11.2 Midwives delivering at home who had delivered fewer than five home births in the last year by regions (NBTF Home Births Survey 1994)

to give birth at home, were included in the remaining (39%). In some areas, these groups provide continuity of care to women with specific needs, such as women with previous problems of neonatal death, or a baby born with congenital abnormality. Also in need of specialist midwifery

Table 11.1 Midwives' attendance of home births in the past year by regions (NBTF Home Births Survey 1994)

	Midwives' attendance							
	0–5		6–10		11–20		21–50	
Region	*n*	%	*n*	%	*n*	%	*n*	%
Northern	105	95.5	5	4.5	0	—	0	—
Yorkshire	158	81.9	34	17.6	1	0.5	0	—
Trent	189	83.6	30	13.3	7	3.1	0	—
East Anglia	220	65.1	90	26.6	28	8.3	0	—
North West Thames	164	49.1	86	25.7	57	17.1	27	8.1
North East Thames	148	57.8	42	16.4	30	11.7	36	14.1
South East Thames	151	33.6	155	34.6	88	19.6	55	12.2
South West Thames	159	60.5	63	24.0	18	6.8	23	8.7
Wessex	132	50.8	39	15.0	60	23.0	29	11.2
Oxford	216	76.8	46	16.4	19	6.8	0	—
South Western	226	45.4	127	25.5	136	27.3	9	1.8
West Midlands	272	84.2	43	13.3	6	1.9	2	0.6
Mersey	80	76.2	25	23.8	0	—	0	—
North Western	181	76.4	48	20.2	8	3.4	0	—
Northern Ireland	23	100.0	0	—	0	—	0	—
Scotland	178	90.4	16	8.1	3	1.5	0	—
Wales	209	76.3	58	21.2	7	2.5	0	—
Total UK	2811	64.3	907	20.8	468	10.7	181	4.2

care were refugee women or women who have experienced rape or abuse. Representatives of all these groups participated in this study.

In the recent report of the Confidential Enquiry into Stillbirths and Neonatal Deaths[6], the proportion of deaths in home births did differ significantly from hospital births and avoidable factors such as insufficient skills and poor risk recognition were identified. The recommendation in that report was that there should be training programmes for both community-based and hospital-based professionals in the management of complications and neonatal resuscitation.

Benefits and difficulties of home births

Some reported particular situations which had proved to be difficult when the parents refused to accept advice, examination, or specific aspects of care. One midwife commented:

I am happy to undertake home births. It saddened me when, even from booking, this lady seemed to reject midwifery care which was probably due to her fear of hospitals. Her antenatal period was uneventful. However, when she became postmature, she seemed oblivious to our anxiety relating to such and to the well-being of herself and her baby. She was Caesarean sectioned within one hour of our struggle to get her into hospital (thick meconium, late decelerations on the CTG, no cervical dilatation, Supervisor of Midwives involvement).

A midwife's satisfaction in her job is greatly increased when she is able to provide continuity of care, has a high level of autonomy and is able to make use of all her skills. This has been shown in previous studies on Home Births[7] and Team Midwifery[8] and was also reported in many of the comments in this survey.

I find them [home births] extremely rewarding and gain a great deal of job satisfaction particularly when you have been the sole care provider.

Some midwives, however, found that the benefits of having greater autonomy and the flexibility to provide continuity of care did not outweigh the disadvantages such as the lack of support from other professionals at the place of birth.

Further disadvantages were the overtime with no extra pay and often no time off in lieu and being on-call throughout the 24 h. The Department of Health, catalysed by the intervention of the last Secretary of State, has spent much effort in improving the duty conditions for junior hospital doctors in the last 3 years. Perhaps a parallel effort for midwives doing home births could lead to a boost in their morale. Some 7.5% of midwives were employed on a scale lower than a G grade although performing the same role. Comments were also made about the stress caused to both mother and midwife when the GP not only refused to provide support for the home birth but also criticized the woman's decision to opt for her choice. Further stress was caused when the midwife, in order to provide continuity of care, promised the woman that she would be available for the birth at all times.

I was on unpaid 'standby' for the last 3 weeks – this is tiring and stressful. There is no formal provision for two midwives – only one is on call per day. I was on my day off and had plans made which I gave up for her delivery. My husband is understanding but being available is very disruptive.

Team midwifery was in operation in many areas to provide the advantages of continuity of care to a small caseload of women without experiencing the disadvantage of the midwife working in isolation. In this system, both moral and practical support may be provided to the midwife by her peers within the teams. In the Institute of Manpower Study[8], which examined the implications of team midwifery for midwives, it was found that in most areas each team midwife, whether the post is graded E, F, or G, has the responsibility of providing total care to the women allocated to her. Extra responsibilities of team leadership and management are then added to the G grade post. Monitoring, teaching and assessing are included in both F and G grade posts. In practice, however, some E grade midwives were asked or expected to extend their role when the F and G grades were not on duty.

In a study where 30 hospital and community midwives in the West Midlands were interviewed to examine their views on home birth, it was reported that the lower grades were associated with less experience and less confidence in caring for women in labour at home as would be expected[9]. In the NBTF 1994 study this was one of the regions with a high proportion of midwives having been at five or fewer home births in the previous year (Table 11.1). In the West Midlands study, none of the midwives, whatever the grade, wanted to give commitment to 24-h call, although the majority were in favour of all women having choice in their place of birth.

Conclusion

Many midwives stated that the only way to learn about home birth is to witness and undertake them and yet almost two-thirds of the respondents had attended fewer than six in the past year. Training in specific skills, (e.g. resuscitation and the siting of intravenous cannulae) would give the midwife confidence to deal with some emergencies but she also needs the support of experienced midwives and some obstetrical practitioners with a special interest in home births to enable her to deal with difficult situations which can occur in the home.

Midwives enjoy an increased level of job satisfaction when providing intrapartum care in the woman's home. This is due to their ability to provide continuity of care, have flexible working patterns and more autonomy. The disadvantages, however, which accompany these benefits for the midwives are highlighted – 24-h on-call, unpaid overtime and the lack of support from peers and medical staff.

IMPLICATIONS FOR DOCTORS

The general practitioner

The doctors in the front line for home births are the GPs. While the midwives carry the major load, a GP can be called to attend in labour for emergencies or if booked, could be present at some time in labour or delivery. We do not know from our survey how many were on call; there is in theory always a practitioner available for emergency maternity work in each practice area. From the answers to question B13 in the midwives' questionnaire (Chapter 4) it would seem that the lead professional at the delivery was a GP in only 33 (1%) cases but in another 537 (12%) cases, the GP was present during the delivery. This, however, does not include the large number of GPs who were on call or attended in the home at some time during labour at an earlier stage but not at delivery itself.

Less likely to be involved in domiciliary births are the hospital teams of obstetricians, paediatricians and anaesthetists; they provide emergency cover for problems which may arise.

With the decline in home births, the interest of the GPs has diminished. They are very active in the antenatal field where they can be the gatekeeper of the antenatal service whether the actual hands-on care is provided by themselves, by midwives or by hospital teams of doctors. The days when difficult deliveries were performed in the home have long gone; the practitioners who were experienced in forceps in the soft domestic bed or in unexpected breech delivery have mostly given up obstetrics or retired completely from general practice. The new generation of GP coming along has been exposed to hospital obstetrics and has seen the operative procedures performed under hospital conditions. They are therefore loath to try to repeat these in the community and so have not the training or experience for work in the domiciliary sector.

As well as a perceived lack of expertise, the shadow of a medicolegal enquiry into obstetrical events when things do not go as the parents expected looms over both hospital and GP. In hospital, vicarious liability covers the medicolegal expenses of hospital staff caring for NHS patients so that the Trust authorities carry the financial and moral burden of medical litigation. This is not so in general practice and so the GP may feel the risk is not worth the hassle as well as possible increased defence organizations subscriptions. At the time of publication medicolegal actions being taken in the UK relating to GPs at home births are rare but the potential for action is there.

The effect of home deliveries on the total practice work-load is another negative factor. As well as the whole problem of night and weekend hours with compensatory rest after extra work, a home birth coming in the middle of a morning surgery of pre-fixed appointments, makes time management difficult.

Financial considerations of a GP involved with home births must be considered for they exist as a continuum from the past. A certain proportion of the practice income may come from the understanding that GPs will be available for and attend intrapartum events. It is hard to change the rules of economic income in the middle of a discussion. However, this nettle must be grasped and compensation made for GPs loss of past contracted earnings if they do not want to participate in the domiciliary delivery load. The new White paper[10] on the future of general practice may provide an opportunity to consider this matter afresh and lead to new contractual arrangements.

If those in general practice still wish to do domiciliary obstetrics, then preliminary and continuing training must be provided. This is very different from the team approach in hospital where there is always someone to call if you are in trouble. Several obstetricians of different levels of experience are available; even consultant obstetricians run into trouble sometimes and they too can always call upon their colleagues. Delivery in the home is different and all of us who used to do domiciliary deliveries have memories of events happening which might have gone otherwise had the deliveries been in an equipped and staffed hospital. Possibly it is these blacker memories of a few ill-fated home births that have influenced senior hospital obstetricians to stand out against domiciliary deliveries. They are remembering these sad events; maybe following a survey of this nature, showing that the risks of *booked* home delivery are low, a change in senior obstetricians' thoughts may follow. The postpartum haemorrhage rates and needs for infant intubation were very low in the 1994 survey (Chapters 5 and 6). If this is pointed out to the women making decisions about planned home delivery, they and their obstetricians may think more positively about this choice. This was well demonstrated in the results of decisions of pregnant women after non-directional counselling[11] but in the NBTF study women were prepared to take very little risk.

If GPs are to take a revised role in home births, a clear pattern of shared management must be worked out locally with the relevant midwives and with the hospital doctors in support. The concept of the lead professional needs clarifying and it seems common sense that it will often be the midwife[12,13]. Education and training for home delivery should begin with the medical student and continue for those doctors wishing to enter family medicine looking after home births. The senior house officer training for those going into general practice obstetrics should differ from that of senior house officer who are going to specialize in obstetrics[12,13] with experience in the community.

Hospital doctors

In the 1930s when half the births were at home, obstetrical flying squads started to provide the presence of hospital doctors and equipment to help in a home delivery in time of trouble. As the number of home births fell these emergency services atrophied. With the more economically driven medical staff levels found in the hospital now, one cannot lose an experienced obstetric registrar from the hospital where they may be overseeing several women in a labour ward in order to care for one woman outside. This reflected in the fact that in the answer to question B13 in the midwives' questionnaire not a single hospital doctor is recorded as being present among some 4500 births (Chapter 4). These data do not include the women who were transferred to hospital before or in labour when obviously hospital doctors took their relevant part in the care.

Even less likely was it that the paediatrician would be present at a home delivery although he was sometimes called out afterwards. Most emergencies of the newborn require instant attention, so such a call after the event would be too late for resuscitation of the newborn child who does not start breathing.

Anaesthetists tend to stay close to the hospital; the only three epidural or spinal anaesthetics recorded (question B7 of the midwives' questionnaire) were not associated with labour. No general anaesthetics are recorded in the home in the 1994 survey.

Implications for the hospital doctors of a continued increasing home birth service are not great if the expansion continues at its present rate. The provision of emergency beds for those who have to be transferred from home in late pregnancy or in labour must continue and experienced staff must be available to deal with these problems. This is very probably inside the current provisions for work-load at the moment and in the near future.

The position of hospital obstetricians going out to see people in domiciliary settings is changing rapidly. The flying squads have mostly gone, being replaced by experienced paramedics in the ambulance service performing resuscitation and bringing the woman into hospital. This will probably cover the majority of old flying squad calls but there still might be the need for an occasional help in the home. If this means extra staff then Health Authorities must persuade purchasers who wish to provide a home delivery service to allocate the money for this in order to provide an adequate service.

The position of the paediatrician and obstetrical anaesthetist mirrors this. Very rarely would an anaesthetist be expected to go out of the hospital. The paediatrician may be called but not so much for resuscitation as for elective care of the baby with an unusual and unexpected problem who could not easily be brought to the hospital.

Conclusions

If home births continue at the same level or even with the modest expansion extrapolated from data of the last few years, the implications for doctors mostly involve a rethink of the position of the General Practitioner Obstetrician (GPO). Those interested must be trained in domiciliary obstetrics not hospital obstetrics. They must be allowed time in the practice schedule for unplanned absence as well as the usual time taken for deliveries. Financial rewards for general practitioner obstetrics must be reviewed and the recent opportunity provided by the Department of Health for discussion with the British Medical Association should be grasped.

In the hospital, emergency care for problems must continue. Some 16% of booked home deliveries were transferred to hospital beds (40% of primiparae). Trained doctors in all relevant disciplines must be available in emergency rotas even if this would mean including compensating rest time after long hours of broken sleep.

The professional organizations (Royal Colleges of Midwives, General Practitioners, Obstetricians and Gynaecologists, Anaesthetists and Paediatricians) in co-operative action must lay down guide-lines for their members. The British Medical Association should take a lead in negotiating future recommendations about fees for a realistic general practitioner service providing care for and attending home births. Thus those who really do it are properly rewarded and less monies are spent on the ghost of a traditional service.

Despite some assertions about the value of obstetric involvement in normal labour[14] the most clearly defined role for obstetricians is in the care of women with complicated pregnancies and labour[15]. Such an experience and training may lead to a distorted impression of risk. During a night on duty an obstetric registrar may sleep through many normal deliveries conducted by midwives only to be called to the labour ward for a postpartum haemorrhage or to confirm and deal with fetal distress.

Undergraduate and postgraduate examinations in Obstetrics tend to emphasize complications, risks and adverse outcomes. The ultimate effect of this training and experience is to leave most obstetricians with a distorted concept of risk.

Adverse outcomes such as perinatal deaths and cases of massive haemorrhage are the subject of regular formal audit in most units with the object of identifying avoidable factors. At a local level, such audits are conducted on the basis of observational data only, with little attempt to look at avoidable factors among controls. Both consultants and trainees are encouraged to be self-critical in these circumstances. The triennial Reports of the Confidential Enquiry into Maternal Mortality in UK is read assiduously by all obstetricians and should be by all GPO and practising midwives.

This background may help to explain why the concept of home birth poses such an immense challenge to many obstetricians. To admit that, in well-selected cases within reasonable access of a maternity unit, the risks of home birth are low seems to undermine the collective *raison d'etre* of obstetricians. The problem is further compounded by the higher rate of mortality and morbidity associated with unplanned home birth and the skewed impression of home birth generated by the invisibility of successful home births to the obstetrician. The best possible remedy for this is the ready availability of good quality data so that risks and probabilities can be discussed in a dispassionate, actuarial fashion.

The risks of obstetricians adopting a rigid position with respect to home births are obvious. A blanket opposition to all home births may result in high-risk women attempting to deliver at home, while a reputation for objectivity may make it easier for a woman unsuitable for home birth to accept advice against it. A tolerant attitude will also encourage women and their midwives to transfer early to hospital care when a complication arises during home birth. We should weigh up the evidence of risk for any individual, setting against background data such as this report provides. From this, evidence-based advice can be offered.

IMPLICATIONS FOR HEALTH AUTHORITIES

It is likely that the trend of an increasing number of women wishing for and planning home births will increase. In 1994, 1.8% of women achieved a home birth; probably a third of these were unbooked. Among the booked women, one should allow antenatal facilities for another 20% to include those who planned to deliver at home but were transferred to hospital late in pregnancy; hence the proportion of women for which the Health Authority must cater financially is currently about 2%. Extrapolating the trend shown in Figure 1.2 (Chapter 1) this proportion could rise to about 4% by the year 2000 and theoretically 7% by 2005. All predictions of health needs suffer from many unaccountable variables and so there is little point in speculating on health predictions further than 10 years ahead and even inside that time a variance as much as 50% may occur.

As Table 4.2 shows in Chapter 4 the regional variation of domiciliary obstetrics is enormous. The regions have now devolved to local Health Authorities and Trusts inside those old regional boundaries; these smaller units have taken up the financial planning for their own areas. Perhaps central Health Departments for the four home kingdoms may be expected to take some part in finding extra finance from Treasury if the momentum for home births grows. The results of this survey show consistently that dissatisfaction of women is mostly with the facilities and environment which the Health Authorities cannot afford to improve and so have to allow to continue in the home and hospital maternity system. It is not with the midwives and doctors who run it, often trying to maintain standards under poor conditions.

The comments in the survey carry a strong implication that Health Authorities must get more money from the purchasers for proper objective health education about home births. Well-meaning but biased accounts from both the antagonists and protagonists of home births do not help the women. Objective information must be presented in an acceptable way to women of different age groups, different educational backgrounds and speaking different languages. Proportions and needs of all these subgroups vary from one Health Authority area to another.

Trusts should be responsible for catalysing the preparation of protocols between midwives, GPs and hospitals. Whilst the detailed professional work will be done by the doctors and midwives, the Trusts should be the catalyst for these publications and provide the right facilities for their completion and proper promulgation. The provision of budgets to take on liaison work between the professionals as well as work on the interface of women and the professionals will be required.

The Health Authorities must make plans to provide enough doctors and midwives who are willing to attend home births. The problems of irregular hours of work must be grasped. Can we provide enough individual midwives with enough experience to give continuity of care throughout a whole labour which may be prolonged? What has been done for junior hospital doctors' hours of service must be done for midwives in the domiciliary field. The use of team midwifery and case-load practices may be encouraged for this is a partial answer to the personalization requested by some women now delivered. This survey has shown, however, that the ideal of delivery by a known midwife who did the antenatal care is not foremost in the minds of many women compared with the ability to be at home and have a choice. It is probable that the inability to provide two G grade midwives in homes for labour care will be as much one of the lack of professional availability as financial restraint.

With the atrophy of the hospital obstetrical flying squads, Health Authorities must ensure rapid and thorough training of the paramedics in resuscitation and transportation of pregnant or labouring women and their babies. In many parts of the country this has been well done already but some Health Authorities are lagging behind and not providing funds or teaching facilities. By the same token they must provide a transport service which is available speedily to take the paramedics to the home and bring the woman and baby to hospital if necessary.

During the next decade no reduction of the hospital obstetrical and midwifery service can take place. Even if as many as the suggested 7% of births are in the home in the next decade, there still will be more than 90% of women who go to hospital as well as the emergencies that arrive from the 7% planning home deliveries. Increased shift to the home sector will not be enough to make any noticeable cut-back of hospital obstetric facilities.

CONCLUSION

The outlook is not gloomy from the Health Authorities' point of view. They should provide fair and unbiased information for the women and then ensure the service is kept at a well-staffed level for those who want to use it. This is not to be an enormous financial burden in the next decade but is one which must be budgeted for in advance with purchasers after local agreement with the local professionals and women's consumer organizations and paying cognizance to advice from the Royal Colleges of Midwives, General Practitioners, Obstetricians and Gynaecologists, Paediatricians, and the British Medical Association on this matter.

REFERENCES

1. MIDIRS and The NHS Centre for Reviews and Dissemination (1996). *Informed Choice Initiative*
2. Enkin, M., Keirse, J.N.C., Renfrew, M.J. and Neilson, J.P. (1995). *A Guide To Effective Care in Pregnancy and Childbirth.* (Oxford: Oxford University Press)
3. Cronk, M. (1995). Are midwives prepared for the Home Birth challenge? *MIDIRS Midwif. Dig.*, **5**, 227–9
4. Department of Health. (1993). *Changing Childbirth Part 1: Report of the Expert Maternity Group.* (London: HMSO)
5. Floyd, L. (1995). Community midwives views and experience of home birth. *Midwifery,* **11**, 3–9
6. Department of Health. (1995). *Confidential Enquiry into Stillbirths and Deaths in Infancy – 1993 Annual Report*, Parts 1 & 2. (London: HMSO)
7. Northern & Yorkshire Regional Health Authority. (1994). *Report on the Northern Region Home Birth Survey 1993*
8. Stock, J. and Wraight, A. (1993). *Developing Continuity of Care in Maternity Services.* (London: Institute of Manpower Studies)
9. Devenish, S. (1995). Home births – the midwife's dilemma. *Modern Midwife,* **5**, 19–21
10. Department of Health. (1996). *The Future of Primary Care Medicine.* (London: HMSO)
11. Thornton, J.G. (1988). Measuring patients' values in reproductive medicine. *Contemp. Rev. Obstet. Gynaecol.*, **1**, 5–12
12. Royal College of General Practitioners. (1995). *The Role of the General Practitioners in Maternity Care*, annual paper 72. (London: RCGP)
13. Royal College of Obstetricians and Gynaecologists & Royal College of General Practitioners. (1995). *General Practitioner Vocational Training in Obstetrics and Gynaecology.* (London: RCGP)
14. O'Driscoll, K., Meagher, D. and Boylan, P. (1993). Role of the doctor. In O'Driscoll, K., Meagher, D. and Boylan, P. (eds.) *Active Management of Labour,* pp. 96–9. (London: Mosby Year Book)
15. Keirse, M.J.N.C. (1989). Interaction between primary and secondary care during pregnancy and childbirth. In Chalmers, I., Enkin, M. and Keirse, M.J.N.C. (eds.) *Effective Care in Pregnancy and Childbirth.* pp. 197–201. (Oxford: Oxford University Press)

12

Recommendations

The recommendations are those of the principle authors of the report, Doctors Chamberlain and Crowley and Ann Wraight, an experienced midwife; they are not of necessity those of the National Birthday Trust Fund (NBTF). For convenience they are divided into sections although many recommendations will overlap one another.

COLLECTION OF DATA

(1)   Maternity information collection and publication is in a poor state and needs more money and thought spent on technology and skills to get accurate, precise and promptly produced data. The Central Health Departments have passed information collection with its problems to the Trusts and Health Authorities. There is difficulty in getting up-to-date statistics from the old Office of Population Censuses and Surveys and now the new Office of National Statistics. The Maternity Hospital Episode system is in gross disarray and fragmentation has led to little interest or funding coming from local sources. Ministers of Health are embarrassed when asked private member questions in the House of Commons for they cannot give comprehensive answers. The whole system needs to be re-examined and improved or consumers and professionals cannot learn what is happening.

(2)   Centrally collected information on home births must differentiate booked from non-booked events. As this report has shown repeatedly, there are large differences between these two groups. So often

233

in the past by keeping the two together, the problems of the latter cloud the data of the former.

(3) The NBTF style of special surveys is a limited method of data collection. Ideally perhaps a randomized controlled trial of home births should be performed but this would be difficult in a subject upon which people hold such strong views before they are even invited to join.

(4) Questionnaire surveys may be the only practical way to do this with a large population but they have the disadvantage of lower response rates. The increases in work and time devoted to local audits take their toll. If questionnaire studies are performed using many observations long preparation time is well repaid in getting extra cover of the population.

(5) The need for local ethical approval from local research ethics committees is difficult in a national survey. There is a need for a National Ethics Committee for country-wide work which can give overall approval. This may then be endorsed locally but more swiftly.

INFORMATION

(1) Women are better educated and are demanding to know more about the maternity service they are planning to use. It behoves the Health Authorities to provide the information for them.

(2) Unbiased information about delivery in various sites must be made available for all women. It must be:

(a) Understandable;

(b) Accurate;

(c) In the language and syntax acceptable to the recipients;

(d) Reflect local facilities and practices.

The data of this survey were collected 2 years after *Changing Childbirth*[1] yet the provision of choice was still lacking, not only as regards place of birth but also with other issues such as position, eating and drinking in labour and methods of pain relief.

(3) It is recommended that data such as this survey and others be correlated by unbiased, knowledgeable professionals and information derived from this be produced with a local slant included, for facilities vary enormously from one Health Authority to another. The details of what is required in a house for a home birth should be told so that women are not surprised at practical things – the untidiness of labour and the limited analgesia available.

(4) The final preparation of totally unbiased information for the consumer may perhaps be done by impartial trained staff such as Public Health Consultants advised by obstetricians, midwives and general practitioners.

(5) The Health Authorities must work locally with doctors and mid-wives to produce protocols for the care of women who give birth at home or those who have to be transferred to hospital. There should be input from Maternity Liaison Committees and consumer organiz-ations. These should be agreed locally as well as with central bodies such as Royal Colleges and professional associations.

SATISFACTION

(1) Health Authorities should note that satisfaction with staff was high among both those who planned and delivered in home and those who planned and delivered in hospital. These are probably two populations who need different services. Whilst the current budget could probably cope with a small expansion of home deliveries, should it rise above 4%, this must be increasingly budgeted for if the purchasers wish that good quality care for home births takes place in their own health district.

(2) It should be noted that the satisfaction was high whether the mid-wife had met the woman before or not. Perhaps the expensive one-to-one ideas thought out theoretically before 1993 might be put to one side if women are perfectly happy with a midwife with whom they feel confident and safe. The compromise of Team Midwifery along with other alternatives such as DOMINO and Birthrooms should be actively considered.

(3) There was much dissatisfaction with the facilities in the wards of hospital stay after delivery. Health Authorities must be reminded

that in this field they are dealing with young healthy people, not ill patients who might accept a different standard in order to be cured.

(4)   Health Authorities should not automatically consider that early discharge from hospital after delivery is the aim for all women. Some would like to stay in for longer and planning must be made for this, running the service for women and their babies and not just for accountants.

(5)   The acceptance of primigravidae for planned home birth may be wished for but it must be remembered that in this study 40% of those so booked had to be transferred to hospital after 37 weeks, many of them in labour. This compares with 11% among the multiparous home booked population. Even here however, 27% of those who had a previous Caesarean section were transferred, twice the background proportion.

THE AMBULANCE SERVICES

(1)   Appropriately trained paramedical support for emergency calls to the home and transport to hospital must be fulfilled swiftly. Some Health Authorities are lagging behind on this, using financial constraints as an excuse to further other areas at the expense of the Home Maternity Service.

(2)   When making plans for domiciliary deliveries, the distance from home to the nearest referring hospital and transportation should be planned to cover all times of the year (e.g. heavy tourist traffic in summer or freezing roads in winter).

THE MIDWIVES

(1)   All midwives and doctors need updating in theoretical and practical skills. This is especially relevant to those assisting with home births because the home can be a very isolated place particularly when troubles occur. Skills in resuscitation, and the placing of intravenous therapy must be mastered. Full cover with mobile telephones is essential to summon aid. If no fixed telephone is available (6% of planned home births in this study) portable telephones should be available. The sharing of equipment between

several midwives may be financially wise but the serious implications of unavailable essential items need to be considered.

(2)   Flexible work patterns for midwives at home births will have to be accepted. This would be difficult for some midwives who have become accustomed to a planned timetable in their week.

(3)   Time off needs to be allocated after long spells have been spent on home deliveries, particularly at night. Similar arrangements should be made for midwives to the ones made recently by Health Authorities for junior hospital doctors.

(4)   We would recommend that midwives (as well as doctors) base their practice more upon research. There is some evidence that this is not so at the moment, for example the suturing of the perineum with catgut is still perpetrated by over half those performing it.

(5)   Perhaps midwives should continue to visit in the postnatal period for longer. Dissatisfaction with an early cut-off point was expressed and the visits of Health Visitors are not viewed in the same light. The implications of this in numbers of midwives in the community sector and financing are enormous but they may be helpful to women having babies.

THE DOCTORS

(1)   General practitioners who are going to take their place in home deliveries need relevant training starting at senior house officer level. Their hospital-based learning needs community supplementation and should be different from that of the senior house officer who is going into career obstetrics. It can still be recognized for the Diploma of the Royal College of Obstetricians and Gynaecologists. Experience must be consolidated by working either with some of the general practitioners who are still interested in home births or by working much more closely with experienced midwives.

(2)   Arrangements are needed to cover unplanned absence from regular duties in general practice if any general practitioner is involved with home births. It includes unexpected absences from a planned surgery with appointments and cover for the day after a night at work attending a home birth.

(3)   The financial rewards for doctors attending home deliveries must be reconsidered. More should be allocated to those who assist at births and attend in labour and perhaps less to those who do ante-natal care only and do not go to the home. The negotiations of the British Medical Association on conditions of service in response to the Department of Health document on the future of primary care[2] may allow a chance for this.

(4)   Consultant obstetricians should read these and other data as they are reported. Opinions about home births can then be based on actual contemporary data rather than on ideas of previous decades. The essential difference between outcomes in booked and unbooked home births needs attention and this should be reflected when making decisions or providing advice about a planned home delivery be it at central, local, or individual level.

REFERENCES

1.   Department of Health. (1993). *Changing Childbirth.* (London: HMSO)
2.   Department of Health. (1996). *The Future of Primary Care Medicine.* (London: HMSO)

Appendices – 1994 Survey Questionnaires

National Birthday Trust

1994 Enquiry into Home Births

APPENDIX I

NATIONAL BIRTHDAY TRUST

1994 ENQUIRY INTO HOME BIRTHS

To the midwife caring for the woman who planned to give birth at home.

Dear Colleague,

BACKGROUND TO THE SURVEY

Discussions continue about the wishes of women to deliver where they choose and the relative safety of home and hospital birth (Changing Childbirth 1993); there are still few real facts about the different experiences in the two places. The National Birthday Trust is conducting a National Survey to collect data from both consumers and professionals to learn more about home births.

The main aim of the study is to collect information on every birth which, at 37 weeks gestation, is planned at home. In order to compare that information with a planned hospital birth, a woman with a background similar to the home birth mother needs to be identified.

YOUR INVOLVEMENT IN THE STUDY

I ask for your help with the relevant questionnaires and also to distribute forms to the appropriate women. The study is entirely voluntary but I hope that you and the women will agree to take part because the greater the response, the more valid the findings.

If a woman is planning to give birth to her baby at home under your care during 1994, please tell her about the study when you see her at about 37 weeks gestation. Give her the pink questionnaire and ask her to complete it after she has had the baby. A pre-paid envelope is enclosed so she can return it directly to me.

You then need to identify another woman in your area who, at 37 weeks gestation, has booked to have her baby in hospital around the same time and has a similar background e.g. similar age group and parity. Such controls should be women who would fulfil ideal criteria for home birth.

If she is happy to take part, attach the enclosed sticker to the notes and explain to her that the midwife who cares for her in labour will give her a blue questionnaire to complete after she has had her baby.

Now that you have got agreement from a woman about to have a home birth and a matching woman about to have a hospital birth, please pass their names and EDD on to your Supervisor of Midwives so that they can be entered into the study.

Once the babies have been born, a questionnaire needs to be completed by the two midwives who were present at the births i.e. home (green questionnaire) and hospital (yellow questionnaire). If a multiple birth occurs, please Xerox the questionnaire and complete the relevant details for the second birth.

If there is no woman booked to have her baby in the hospital within a four week period of the home birth, please do not exclude the woman who has a

1

home birth but complete the appropriate questionnaires and return.

If the baby is stillborn or dies soon after birth, I would be grateful if you would still complete your form. In previous studies, women whose baby died have indicated that they still want to relate their experiences; if you feel that it is appropriate, contact your Supervisor of Midwives who will give you the relevant questionnaire for the woman to complete.

CONFIDENTIALITY

All the information you give will be fully confidential. When the forms are returned to the survey office, all personal and geographical details will be replaced with a survey code and from then on the questionnaires will have a number only.

I would be grateful if you could complete the form as soon after the birth as possible and return it to the Supervisor of Midwives who is co-ordinating the collection of the questionnaires in your district.

I appreciate the time this consumes and I thank you for your committment to this national enquiry.

Ann Wraight

Six weeks after the delivery, a random sample of women will be sent a second short questionnaire so that any shift in attitudes and any problems experienced can be identified in both groups.

The following information is therefore required to enable the research team to contact the woman at home.

When this form reaches the survey office, this page will be detached so that the questionnaire is rendered anonymous and cannot be traced to individuals.

Woman's Name _____

Woman's Address _____

_____

postcode _____

Health Authority/Board/Trust _____

Address where baby was born if not the above:

_____

_____

postcode _____

FOR OFFICE USE ONLY

2

How to fill in this questionnaire:

Most questions can be answered by ticking the box or boxes which apply. Please ignore the numbers in or beside the boxes. They are to help me analyse the answers.

Sometimes I would like you to fill in a number in the box(es), and in few cases I would like you to write in your answer in your own words.

Go from one question to the next unless the box you have ticked tells you otherwise. In this way you will miss out questions which do not apply to you.

Please feel free to write in extra comments if you would like to give me more information.

Ann Wraight.

A.   **DESCRIPTIVE DATA ABOUT THE WOMAN**

1.   PAST PREGNANCIES (24 weeks gestation and above):

Year	Site of delivery e.g.home/ hospital	Method of delivery	Gestation	Outcome live/ stillbirth	Birthweight (gm)

PRESENT PREGNANCY :

2.   At what stage of gestation did the booking take place?   Weeks ☐

3.   Did you attend the woman during her pregnancy?   Yes ☐   No ☐

4.   If yes, how many antenatal visits were done by you?   Number ☐

5.   Was an ultrasound scan (not Doppler) performed in pregnancy?   Yes ☐   No ☐

6.   Did you refer the woman directly for the scan?   Yes ☐   No ☐

7.   Was antenatal CTG performed?   Yes ☐   No ☐

8.   Were any other special tests/investigations performed?   Yes ☐   No ☐
     e.g. amniocentesis, Doppler

9.   If yes, please specify _____

10. Did you experience any difficulty referring the woman for special tests/investigations?   Yes ☐   No ☐

11. If yes, please explain what these difficulties were_____

FOR OFFICE USE ONLY

_____ (1-3)
_____ (4-7)
__01__ (8-9)

_____ (10-16)

_____ (17-23)

_____ (24-30)

_____ (31-37)

_____ (38-44)

_____ (45-46)

_____ (47)

_____ (48-49)

_____ (50)

_____ (51)

_____ (52)

_____ (53)

_____ (54)
_____ (55)
_____ (56)

_____ (57)

_____ (58)
_____ (59)
_____ (60)

3

242

GREEN QUESTIONNAIRE

12. Did any of the following complications occur in pregnancy? (Tick any that apply).

Hypertensive disease	Cardiac disease
Diabetes	Antepartum haemorrhage
Mental illness	Intrauterine growth retardation
Pre-eclampsia/PIH	Other

(specify) _____

_____ (61-62)
_____ (63-64)
_____ (65-66)
_____ (67-68)

_____ (69)

13. PLACE OF BIRTH (Tick one box only in each column) :

Intended place of birth   Actual place of birth

1. Home
2. GP unit
3. Midwife led care
4. GP bed
5. Consultant bed
6. Ambulance
7. Other

(specify) _____

_____ (70-71)

_____ (72)

14. PROFESSIONAL SUPPORT
Please specify in each column the number of people who attended the woman during pregnancy, labour and delivery.

_____ (1-3)
_____ (4-7)
__02__ (8-9)

	Pregnancy (Specify no.)	Labour (Specify no.)	Delivery (Specify no.)
Known midwife - community			
hospital			
independent			
Other midwife			
Own GP			
Other GP			
SHO			
Registrar/Senior Reg.			
Consultant			
Other			

(specify) _____

_____ (10-13)
_____ (14-17)
_____ (18-21)
_____ (22-25)
_____ (26-29)
_____ (30-33)
_____ (34-37)
_____ (38-41)
_____ (42-45)
_____ (46-49)

_____ (50)

B. **LABOUR**

_____ (51)

1. Was the labour induced?   Yes ☐   No ☐

_____ (1-3)
_____ (4-7)
__03__ (8-9)

2. When did each stage begin? (Please give date and time, use 24 hour clock).

1st stage   _ / _ / _   Date   Time
2nd stage   _ / _ / _   Date   Time
3rd stage   _ / _ / _   Date   Time

_____ (10-19)
_____ (20-29)
_____ (30-39)

3. When did the 3rd stage end? (Please give date and time)

_ / _ / _   Date   Time

_____ (40-49)

4. When did you arrive at the house/take over her care in labour? (Please give date and time)

_ / _ / _   Date   Time

_____ (50-59)

_____ (60)

5. Had the woman completed a written plan of her wishes for labour?   Yes ☐   No ☐

_____ (61)

6. If plan was not followed, please specify the main reason _____

4

GREEN QUESTIONNAIRE

7. Pain relief used (Tick any that apply)

None	☐	Relaxation/breathing exercises	☐
Entonox	☐	TENS	☐
Meptazinol	☐	Acupuncture	☐
Pethidine	☐	Homeopathy	☐
Diamorphine/Morphine	☐	Aromatherapy	☐
Epidural	☐	Massage	☐
Spinal	☐	Warm water	☐
General Anaesthetic	☐	Other	☐

(specify) _____

_____ (62-63)
_____ (64-65)
_____ (66-67)
_____ (68-69)
_____ (70-71)
_____ (72-73)
_____ (74-75)
_____ (76-77)
_____ (78)
_____ (79)
_____ (1-3)

8. Were the forewaters ruptured artificially?   Yes ☐   No ☐

_____ (4-7)
__04__ (8-9)

9. If yes, what was the cervical dilatation?   ☐☐ cm

10. What position was adopted for delivery (Tick one box only).

_____ (10-11)

1. Propped up in bed	☐	2. Lithotomy	☐
3. Supine with lateral tilt	☐	4. All fours	☐
5. Sitting	☐	6. Standing	☐
7. Birth chair	☐	8. Lateral	☐
9. Supine	☐	10. Squatting	☐
11. Other	☐		

_____ (12-13)

(specify)_____

_____ (14)

11. Did the birth take place in water?   Yes ☐   No ☐

_____ (15)

12. Method of delivery (Tick one box only).

_____ (16)

Spontaneous -		Assisted -	
1. occipito anterior	☐	5. forceps	☐
2. occipito posterior	☐	6. vacuum extraction	☐
3. breech	☐	7. Caesarean Section	☐
4. face	☐	8. Other	☐

_____ (17)

(specify) _____

13. Personnel present at time of birth.

	Who delivered the baby? (Tick one box)	Who was the lead professional at the delivery? (Tick one box)	Who else (i.e. staff) were present at the delivery? (Specify the number present in each relevant box)	
E grade midwife	☐	☐	☐	_____ (18-20)
F grade midwife	☐	☐	☐	_____ (21-23)
G grade midwife	☐	☐	☐	_____ (24-26)
H grade midwife	☐	☐	☐	_____ (27-29)
I grade midwife	☐	☐	☐	_____ (30-32)
Independent midwife	☐	☐	☐	_____ (33-35)
Student midwife	☐	☐	☐	_____ (36-38)
GP	☐	☐	☐	_____ (39-41)
Medical student	☐	☐	☐	_____ (42-44)
SHO	☐	☐	☐	_____ (45-47)
Registrar	☐	☐	☐	_____ (48-50)
Senior reg.	☐	☐	☐	_____ (51-53)
Consultant	☐	☐	☐	_____ (54-56)
Anaesthetist	☐	☐	☐	_____ (57-59)
Paediatrician	☐	☐	☐	_____ (60-62)
Ambulance Officer	☐	☐	☐	_____ (63-65)
Other	☐	☐	☐	_____ (66-68)

(specify) _____

_____ (69)

5

GREEN QUESTIONNAIRE

14. Management of 3rd stage. (Tick any that apply) :

      Physiological

      Controlled cord traction

      Manual removal of placenta

      Syntometrine/Ergometrine

      Syntocinon

      Other

      (specify) _____

      (1-3)
      (4-7)
      05 (8-9)
      (10)
      (11)
      (12)
      (13)
      (14)
      (15)
      (16)

15. Estimated blood loss   ml   (17-20)

16. Perineal damage. (Tick any that apply) :

      None

      1st degree tear

      2nd degree tear

      3rd degree tear

      Episiotomy

      Vaginal tear

      Cervical tear

      (21)
      (22)
      (23)
      (24)
      (25)
      (26)
      (27)

17. Who repaired the tear/episiotomy? (Tick one box only) :

    1. Midwife who delivered baby   2. GP

    3. Other midwife   4. SHO

    5. Registrar   6. Consultant

    7. Other

      (specify) _____

      (28)
      (29)

18. What suture material was used? (Tick any that apply) :

    Catgut   Dexon

    Silk   Dexon/vicryl

    Other

      (specify) _____

      (30-31)
      (32-33)
      (34)
      (35)

19. When did the repair take place? (Please give date and time)

    Date   _ / _ / _   Time   (36-45)

20. Did any complications occur in labour which have not already been mentioned?

        Yes   No

      (46)
      (47)
      (48)

21. If yes, please specify _____ (49)

C. **BABY**

1. Was the baby: Livebirth   Stillbirth   Neonatal death   (50)

2. What was the gestation?   weeks   (51-52)

3. What was the birthweight?   gm   (53-56)

4. What were the Apgar scores?   1 minute   5 minutes   (57-60)

5. Was the baby resuscitated?   Yes   No   (61)

6

6. If yes, what resuscitation was required? (Tick any that apply).

    Aspiration   ☐
    Bag and mask
    Intubation

_____ (62)
_____ (63)
_____ (64)

7. If yes, who resuscitated the baby? (Tick any that apply).

    Midwife   ☐   GP   ☐
    Paediatrician   Obstetrician
    Anaesthetist   Other

                 (specify) _____

_____ (65-66)
_____ (67-68)
_____ (69-70)

_____ (71)

8. Were there any birth injuries?   Yes ☐   No ☐

_____ (72)

9. If yes, please specify _____

_____ (73)

10. Were there any congenital abnormalities?   Yes ☐   No ☐

_____ (74)
_____ (75)

11. If yes, please specify _____

_____ (1-3)
_____ (4-7)
__06___ (8-9)

....

D. **EQUIPMENT AND TRAINING**

1. Which of the following items were available for the home birth? (Tick any that apply).

    Telephone   ☐   IV infusion set   ☐
    Radiopager   IV fluids
    Sonicaid   Neonatal Narcan
    Entonox   Oxygen for mother
    Bag and mask   Oxygen for baby
    Intubation equipment

_____ (10)
_____ (11-12)
_____ (13-14)
_____ (15-16)
_____ (17-18)
_____ (19-20)
_____ (21-22)
_____ (23-24)
_____ (25-26)
_____ (27)

2. Have you received any _theoretical_ training relating to home birth in the past two years?   Yes ☐   No ☐

_____ (28)

3. Have you received any _practical_ training relating to home birth in the past two years?   Yes ☐   No ☐

_____ (29)

4. With how many home births have you assisted in the past year?   Number ☐☐

_____ (30-31)

Thank you very much for completing this form. Please make any additional comments which you feel are important. If the mother had to be transferred for hospital care, please give further details on the next page.

_____ (32)

GREEN QUESTIONNAIRE

E   **PLANNED HOME BIRTHS**

Please complete this page if the woman had to be <u>transferred from home for hospital care after 37 weeks</u> <u>gestation</u> whether for maternal or fetal/neonatal reasons.

1.   Method of transfer (Tick one box only).

    1. Obstetric flying squad
    2. Neonatal flying squad
    3. Ambulance with paramedics
    4. Ambulance with midwife
    5. Ambulance with midwife and paramedics
    6. Car   _____ (33)
    7. Helicopter/plane
    8. Other

    (specify) _____ _____ (34)

2.   When was the call for assistance made?   Date   _ / _ / _   time [   ]   _____ (35-44)

3.   When did help arrive?   Date   _ / _ / _   time [   ]   _____ (45-54)

4.   What care was initiated before transfer? _____   _____ (55)
    _____ (56)
    _____   _____ (57)

5.   Did you accompany the woman to hospital?   Yes [   ]   No [   ]   _____ (58)

6.   How long did the journey take?   [   ] hours [   ] minutes   _____ (59-62)

7.   What were the reasons for transfer? (Tick any that apply)

    a) mother
    Prolonged labour [   ]   Malpresentation [   ]   _____ (63-64)
    Antepartum haemorrhage [   ]   Postpartum haemorrhage [   ]   _____ (65-66)
    Retained placenta [   ]   3rd degree tear [   ]   _____ (67-68)
    Dystocia [   ]   Other [   ]   _____ (69-70)

    (specify)_____   _____ (71)

    _____ (1-3)
    b) baby   _____ (4-7)
    Fetal distress [   ]   Cord prolapse [   ]   _07__ (8-9)
    Low birth weight [   ]   Asphyxia [   ]
    Birth trauma [   ]   Congenital abnormality [   ]
    Intra uterine growth [   ]   Other [   ]   _____ (10-11)
         retardation   _____ (12-13)
    (specify) _____   _____ (14-15)

8.   What was the management in hospital? (Tick any that apply)   _____ (16-17)
    _____ (18)

    a) mother
    Induction of labour [   ]   Augmentation of labour [   ]   _____ (19-20)
    Assisted delivery [   ]   Caesarean Section [   ]   _____ (21-22)
    Manual removal of placenta [   ]   Blood transfusion [   ]   _____ (23-24)
    Repair of laceration [   ]   Other [   ]   _____ (25-26)
    _____ (27)
    (specify) _____

    b) baby
    Incubator care [   ]   Respiratory support [   ]   _____ (28-29)
    Surgery [   ]   Blood transfusion [   ]   _____ (30-31)
    Other [   ]   _____ (32)
    _____ (33)
    (specify) _____

8

APPENDIX II

PLANNED HOME BIRTH

WOMAN'S QUESTIONNAIRE

THE NATIONAL BIRTHDAY TRUST

1994 ENQUIRY INTO HOME BIRTHS

CONFIDENTIAL

Please return completed forms to :

Ann Wraight
Midwife Co-ordinator
The National Birthday Trust
Department of Obstetrics & Gynaecology
St George's Hospital Medical School
Cranmer Terrace
London SW17 ORE

PINK QUESTIONNAIRE

Congratulations on the birth of your baby.

I hope that you can spare a few minutes to read this questionnaire and answer a few questions about your labour.

The aim of this survey is to find out about your experiences at the birth of your baby at home. This is a national study and so every woman towards the end of her pregnancy who has planned to have her baby at home in the UK this year is being asked to complete a questionnaire. When a home birth takes place, a woman who has chosen to have her baby in hospital will also be asked to fill in this form so that the births, happening around the same time in the two places, can be compared. Your midwife will also be asked to complete a form about factual information about the birth. If your baby was not born at home as planned, please complete the questionnaire because it is important for me to know what happened.

The information you give is <u>confidential</u>. Your name and address will be replaced by code numbers as soon as the questionnaire reaches the survey office, so please express your feelings freely. When all the results have been analysed, these will be used to determine what plans need to be made in the future regarding place of birth. No information goes back to your midwife or doctor.

When your baby is 6 weeks old, you may receive a second short questionnaire to complete. This will tell me whether you hold the same views about your baby's birth or whether you have changed your mind on some issues.

If you are happy to answer these questions, please do so as soon as possible while the memory of the labour is still fresh in your mind and post the questionnaire back to me. A pre-paid envelope is enclosed for your convenience.

Thank you very much for your help.

Ann Wraight
Midwife Co-ordinator
The National Birthday Trust

....

PERSONAL DETAILS :

NAME : _____

ADDRESS : _____

_____

post code _____

DATE of filling in this form : _____/_____/1994

| FOR OFFICE |
| USE ONLY |
| _____ |
| _____ |

2

PLANNED HOME BIRTHS

How to fill in this questionnaire :

Most questions can be answered by ticking the box or boxes which apply to you. Please ignore numbers in or beside the boxes. They are to help me analyse the answers.

Sometimes I would like you to fill in a number in the box(es), and in a few cases I would like you to write in your answer in your own words.

Go from one question to the next unless the box you have ticked tells you otherwise. In this way you will not have to answer questions which do not apply to you.

Please feel free to write in extra comments if you would like to give me more information.

Ann Wraight

FOR OFFICE USE ONLY

_____ (1-3)
_____ (4-7)
__01__ (8-9)

A **Please fill in the following questions about yourself. It will help me to know what kinds of people the survey represents.**

1. What is your date of birth? ___/___/___   _____ (10-15)

2. How many children do you have apart from this one? Number [ ][ ]   _____ (16-17)

3. To which of these ethnic groups do you belong? (Tick one box only)

1.	White		2.	West Indian	
3.	Indian		4.	Pakistani	
5.	Bangladeshi		6.	African	
7.	Arab		8.	Other	

specify _____   _____ (18)

_____ (19)

4. If English your first language? Yes [ ] No [ ]   _____ (20)

5. If no, how well do you speak English? (Tick one box only)

| 1. | Very well | | 2. | Fairly well | |
| 3. | Not very well | | 4. | Not at all | |

_____ (21)

6. What is your present occupation? (Please write in the job name or type of work. If not working now, write in previous or usual job).

_____   _____ (22)

7. Please write in the job name or type of work of your husband's/partner's present occupation if applicable. If not working now, write in previous or usual job.

_____   _____ (23)

8. If your husband/partner currently working? 1. Yes 2. No 3. Not applicable [ ]   _____ (24)
(Tick one box only)

_____ (25-26)

9. How old were you when you left school or finished full time education?

(enter age in years) [ ][ ]

B.   **YOUR PREGNANCY**

1.   At what stage did you decide to have your baby at home? (Tick one box only)

　　　　1. Before pregnancy ☐　　2. Early pregnancy ☐
　　　　3. Middle pregnancy　　　 4. Late pregnancy

_____ (27)

2.   What was your main reason for choosing to have your baby at home?

_____

_____ (28)

_____

3.   How many of the following people did you speak to about home births? Did they encourage
　　　or discourage you to have your baby at home? (Please tick any box which applies in each row).

	Spoke to	Encouraged me	Discouraged me	
Husband/partner	☐	☐	☐	(29-31)
Children	☐	☐	☐	(32-34)
Mother	☐	☐	☐	(35-37)
Mother-in-law	☐	☐	☐	(38-40)
Other family	☐	☐	☐	(41-43)
Community midwife	☐	☐	☐	(44-46)
Hospital midwife	☐	☐	☐	(47-49)
Independent midwife	☐	☐	☐	(50-52)
GP	☐	☐	☐	(53-55)
Hospital doctor	☐	☐	☐	(56-58)
Health visitor	☐	☐	☐	(59-61)
Friends	☐	☐	☐	(62-64)
Others	☐	☐	☐	(65-67)
				(68)

　　　(specify) _____

4.   If you were discouraged from having a home birth, what was the main reason given?

_____

_____ (69)

_____

5.   Did you have any of the following problems in pregnancy? (Tick any that apply)

_____ (70-71)
_____ (72-73)
_____ (74-75)
_____ (76)

　　　　High blood pressure ☐　　　Pre-eclampsia ☐
　　　　Diabetes　　　　　　　　　　Heart disease
　　　　Vaginal bleeding ☐　　　　　Other ☐
　　　　　　　　　　　　　　　　　　(specify) _____

....

C.   **YOUR LABOUR**

_____ (77)

1.   Did you want to drink any fluids during labour?　　Yes ☐　　No ☐

_____ (78)
_____ (79)

2.   If yes, when did you have something to drink?
　　　(Tick any that apply).　　　　　　Early labour ☐
　　　　　　　　　　　　　　　　　　　 Middle labour
　　　　　　　　　　　　　　　　　　　 Late labour

_____ (80)

_____ (1-3)
_____ (4-7)

3.   Did you want to eat any food during labour?　　Yes ☐　　No ☐

__02__ (8-9)

4.   If yes, when did you have something to eat?
　　　(Tick any that apply).　　　　　　Early labour ☐
　　　　　　　　　　　　　　　　　　　 Middle labour
　　　　　　　　　　　　　　　　　　　 Late labour

_____ (10)

_____ (11)
_____ (12)
_____ (13)

5.   Did you have your baby at home?　　Yes ☐　　No ☐

_____ (14)

4

IF YES PLEASE MOVE ON TO QUESTION 14.

6. If NO, where was your baby born?
    (Tick one box only)
    1. In ambulance
    2. In hospital
    3. Other
       specify _____

_____ (15)

_____ (16)

7. If you had to be admitted to hospital what were the reasons given?

    _____

_____ (17)
_____ (18)

    _____

_____ (19)

8. Did you agree with the reasons given?   Yes [ ]   No [ ]   Don't know [ ]

_____ (20)

9. If no, please explain _____

_____ (21)

    _____

10. Were you familiar with the labour ward?
                        Yes [ ]   No [ ]

_____ (22)

11. How did you find the transfer to the hospital? (Tick one box only)

    1. Very upsetting
    2. Moderately upsetting
    3. Not at all upsetting

_____ (23)

12. Did your midwife continue to look after you in hospital?   Yes [ ]   No [ ]

_____ (24)

13. Was this important to you? (Tick one box only)

    1. Very important
    2. Moderately important
    3. Not very important
    4. Not at all important

_____ (25)

14. The following people may have been with you <u>during your labour</u>. Please say whether or not they were there and whether you were pleased that they were there. (Please tick any box which applies in each row).

	Present during labour	I was pleased they were there	
Husband/partner	[ ]	[ ]	(26-27)
Children	[ ]	[ ]	(28-29)
Mother	[ ]	[ ]	(30-31)
Known midwife	[ ]	[ ]	(32-33)
Other midwife	[ ]	[ ]	(34-35)
Student midwife	[ ]	[ ]	(36-37)
GP	[ ]	[ ]	(38-39)
Obstetrician	[ ]	[ ]	(40-41)
Anaesthetist	[ ]	[ ]	(42-43)
Paediatrician (baby's doctor)	[ ]	[ ]	(44-45)
Student doctor	[ ]	[ ]	(46-47)
Student nurse	[ ]	[ ]	(48-49)
Friends	[ ]	[ ]	(50-51)
Others	[ ]	[ ]	(52-53)

    (specify) _____

_____ (54)

5

15. The following people may have been with you during or <u>at the birth of your</u>
<u>baby</u>. Please say whether or not they were there and whether you were pleased that they
were there. (Please tick any box which applies in each row).

	Present at the birth	I was pleased they were there		
			_____	(1-3)
			_____	(4-7)
			__03__	(8-9)
			_____	(10-11)
Husband/partner			_____	(12-13)
Children			_____	(14-15)
Mother			_____	(16-17)
Known midwife			_____	(18-19)
Other midwife			_____	(20-21)
Student midwife			_____	(22-23)
GP			_____	(24-25)
Obstetrician			_____	(26-27)
Anaesthetist			_____	(28-29)
Paediatrician (baby's doctor)			_____	(30-31)
Student doctor			_____	(32-33)
Student nurse			_____	(34-35)
Friends			_____	(36-37)
Others			_____	(38)

(specify) _____

16. What did you use to help relieve the pain of labour and what did you find helpful? (Please
tick any box which applies in each row).

	Used	Helpful		
None			_____	(39-40)
Relaxation/breathing exercises			_____	(41-42)
Massage			_____	(43-44)
Warm water			_____	(45-46)
TENS			_____	(47-48)
Acupuncture			_____	(49-50)
Homeopathy			_____	(51-52)
Aromatherapy			_____	(53-54)
Injection eg. Pethidine			_____	(55-56)
Epidural			_____	(57-58)
Spinal			_____	(59-60)
Entonox (gas & oxygen)			_____	(61-62)
General Anaesthetic			_____	(63-64)
Other			_____	(65-66)
			_____	(67)

(specify) _____

*NB   IF YOU DID <u>NOT HAVE HOSPITAL CARE</u>, PLEASE MOVE ON TO QUESTION D1

17. What treatment did you need in hospital? (Tick any that apply)

None		Induction of labour		_____	(68-69)
Drip to speed up labour		Forceps/Vacuum delivery		_____	(70-71)
Caesarean Section		Blood transfusion		_____	(72-73)
Removal of placenta		Repair of tear		_____	(74-75)
Other				_____	(76)

(specify)_____

_____ (77)

18. Was the treatment discussed with you?   Yes [   ]   No [   ]

_____ (78)

6

19. What treatment did baby need? (Tick any that apply)

None	Incubator care
Help with breathing	Surgery
Blood transfusion	Other

(specify)_____

_____ (1-3)
_____ (4-7)
__04__ (8-9)
_____ (10-11)
_____ (12-13)
_____ (14-15)

_____ (16)

20. Was the baby's treatment discussed with you?   Yes [ ]   No [ ]

_____ (17)

21. How many days did you stay in hospital?   Days [ ]

_____ (18-19)

22. Did you feel that this was about the right length of time?
(Tick one box only)
1. Yes
2. No, too short
3. No, too long

_____ (20)

23. How many days did your baby stay in hospital?   Days [ ]

_____ (21-22)

24. OTHER COMMENTS :
Please tell us anything you think is important about your admission to hospital.

_____ (23)

....

D. AFTER THE BIRTH OF YOUR BABY

1. Did you experience any of the following problems in the first 48 hours after the birth
of the baby? (Tick any that apply).

Tiredness	Headache
Backache	Painful stitches
Constipation	Piles
Breast problems	Tearfulness
Abnormal vaginal bleeding	Urine infection
Leaking urine	High blood pressure
Other	

(Specify) _____

_____ (24-25)
_____ (26-27)
_____ (28-29)
_____ (30-31)
_____ (32-33)
_____ (34-35)
_____ (36)

_____ (37)

2. How are you feeding your baby? (Please tick one box only).

1. Breast milk only
2. Breast & bottle milk
3. Bottle milk only

_____ (38)

3. Is this how you had planned to feed your baby?   Yes [ ]   No [ ]

_____ (39)

4. When you fed your baby for the first time, how did the baby respond?
(Tick any that apply)

Fed well	Irritable
Not interested	Was sick
Sleepy	Other

(specify) _____

_____ (40-41)
_____ (42-43)
_____ (44-45)
_____ (46)

7

254

5. Were you happy about your decision to have a home birth? (Tick one box only)

    1. Very happy
    2. Moderately happy
    3. Not very happy
    4. Rather unhappy

    _____ (47)

N.B. IF YOU HAD YOUR BABY IN HOSPITAL, MOVE ON TO QUESTION 8.

6. What did you like <u>most</u> about having your baby at home?

    _____

    _____   _____ (48)

7. What did you like <u>least</u> about having your baby at home?

    _____   _____ (49)

    _____

8. How do you feel about the care you received from the midwives at birth? (Tick one box only).

    1. Very satisfied
    2. Satisfied
    3. Dissatisfied
    4. Very dissatisfied
    5. Don't know

    _____ (50)

9. How do you feel about the care you received from the doctors at birth? (Tick one box only).

    1. Very satisfied
    2. Satisfied
    3. Dissatisfied
    4. Very dissatisfied
    5. Don't know
    6. Not applicable

    _____ (51)

10. If you have another baby, where would you choose to give birth? (Tick one box only).

    1. Home
    2. Hospital rather than home
    3. GP unit
    4. Other

    _____ (52)

        (specify) _____   _____ (53)

Thank you very much for completing this form. Please add any other relevant comments.

    _____ (54)

8

255

APPENDIX III

PLANNED HOSPITAL BIRTH

WOMAN'S QUESTIONNAIRE

THE NATIONAL BIRTHDAY TRUST

1994 ENQUIRY INTO HOME BIRTHS

CONFIDENTIAL

Please return completed forms to :

Ann Wraight
Midwife Co-ordinator
The National Birthday Trust
Department of Obstetrics & Gynaecology
St George's Hospital Medical School
Cranmer Terrace
London SW17 0RE

1

BLUE QUESTIONNAIRE

Congratulations on the birth of your baby.

I hope that you can spare a few minutes to read this questionnaire and answer a few questions about your labour.

The aim of this survey is to find out about your experiences at the birth of your baby in hospital. This is a national study and so every woman towards the end of her pregnancy who has planned to have her baby at home in the UK this year is being asked to complete a questionnaire. When a home birth takes place, a woman who has chosen to have her baby in hospital, as you have, will also be asked to fill in this form so that the births, happening around the same time in the two places, can be compared. Your midwife will also be asked to complete a form about factual information about the birth.

The information you give is <u>confidential</u>. Your name and address will be replaced by code numbers as soon as the questionnaire reaches the survey office, so please express your feelings freely. When all the results have been analysed, these will be used to determine what plans need to be made in the future regarding place of birth. No information goes back to your midwife or your doctor.

When your baby is 6 weeks old, you may receive a second short questionnaire to complete. This will tell me whether you hold the same views about your baby's birth or whether you have changed your mind on some issues.

If you are happy to answer these questions, please do so as soon as possible while the memory of the labour is still fresh in your mind and post the questionnaire back to me. A pre-paid envelope is enclosed for your convenience.

Thank you very much for your help.

Ann Wraight
Midwife Co-ordinator
The National Birthday Trust

....

PERSONAL DETAILS :

NAME : _____

ADDRESS : _____

_____

post code _____

DATE of filling in this form : ____ /____ /1994

```
┌──────────────┐
│ FOR OFFICE   │
│ USE ONLY     │
│              │
│ _____     │
│              │
│ _____     │
└──────────────┘
```

2

BLUE QUESTIONNAIRE

<u>PLANNED HOSPITAL BIRTHS</u>

<u>How to fill in this questionnaire :</u>

Most questions can be answered by ticking the box or boxes which apply to you. Please ignore numbers in or beside the boxes. They are to help me analyse the answers.

Sometimes I would like you to fill in a number in the box, and in a few cases I would like you to write in your answer in your own words.

Go from one question to the next unless the box you have ticked tells you otherwise. In this way you will miss out questions which do not apply to you.

Please feel free to write in extra comments if you would like to give me more information.

Ann Wraight

FOR OFFICE
USE ONLY

_____ (1-3)
_____ (4-7)
___01___ (8-9)

A   Please fill in the following questions about yourself. It will help me to know what kinds of people the survey represents.

_____ (10-15)

1.   What is your date of birth?   __/__/__

_____ (16-17)

2.   How many children do you have apart from this one?   Number [   ]

3.   To which of these ethnic groups do you belong? (Tick one box only)

1.	White	[ ]	2.	West Indian	[ ]	
3.	Indian	[ ]	4.	Pakistani	[ ]	
5.	Bangladeshi	[ ]	6.	African	[ ]	
7.	Arab	[ ]	8.	Other	[ ]	

specify _____

_____ (18)

_____ (19)

4.   If English your first language?   Yes [ ]   No [ ]

_____ (20)

5.   If no, how well do you speak English? (Tick one box only)

1.	Very well	[ ]	2.	Fairly well	[ ]
3.	Not very well		4.	Not at all	

_____ (21)

6.   What is your present occupation? (Please write in the job name or type of work. If not working now, write in <u>previous or usual</u> job).

_____

_____ (22)

7.   What is your husband's/partner's present occupation? (Please write in the job name or type of work. If not working now, write in <u>previous or usual</u> job).

_____

_____ (23)

8.   If your husband/partner currently working?   1. Yes   [ ]
(Tick one box only)   2. No
                                   3. Not applicable

_____ (24)

_____ (25-26)

9.   How old were you when you left school or finished full time education?

(enter age in years) [   ]

3

BLUE QUESTIONNAIRE

B. YOUR PREGNANCY

1. At what stage did you decide to have your baby in hospital? (Tick one box only)

    1. Before pregnancy
    2. Early pregnancy
    3. Middle Pregnancy
    4. Late pregnancy

    _____ (30)

2. What was your main reason for choosing to have your baby in hospital?

    _____ (31)

3. How many of the following people did you speak to about where you should have your baby?
    Did they encourage or discourage you to have your baby in hospital? (Please tick any box
    which applies in each row)

	Spoke to	Encouraged me	Discouraged me	
Husband/partner				_____ (32-34)
Children				_____ (35-37)
Mother				_____ (38-40)
Mother-in-law				_____ (41-43)
Other family				_____ (44-46)
Community midwife				_____ (47-49)
Hospital midwife				_____ (50-52)
Independent midwife				_____ (53-55)
GP				_____ (56-58)
Hospital doctor				_____ (59-61)
Health visitor				_____ (62-64)
Friends				_____ (65-67)
Others				_____ (68-70)

    (specify) _____   _____ (71)

4. If you were discouraged from having a hospital birth, what was the **main** reason given?

    _____ (72)

5. Did you consider any alternative to hospital birth?   Yes [   ]   No [   ]

    _____ (73)

6. Were any of the following options discussed with you? (Tick any that apply).

    Homebirth [   ]   DOMINO [   ]   _____ (74-75)
    GP unit   Other   _____ (76-77)
                                                          _____ (78)
                               (specify) _____

                                                          _____ (1-3)
7. Did you have any of the following problems in pregnancy? (Tick any that apply)   _____ (4-7)
                                                                                      __02__ (8-9)
    High blood pressure [   ]   Pre-eclampsia [   ]   _____ (10-11)
    Diabetes   Heart disease   _____ (12-13)
    Vaginal bleeding   Other   _____ (14-15)
                                                            _____ (16)
                               (specify)_____

4

259

C.   YOUR LABOUR

1.   Did you want to drink any fluids during labour?   Yes [ ]   No [ ]   _____ (17)

2.   If yes, when did you want to drink? (Tick any that apply).

                                        Early labour [ ]   _____ (18)
                                      Middle labour [ ]   _____ (19)
                                      Late labour [ ]   _____ (20)

   _____ (21)

3.   Were you allowed to drink within reason what you wanted?   [ ] Yes   [ ] No   _____ (22)

4.   If no, what was the reason? _____

   _____ (23)
   _____

5.   Did you want to eat any food during labour?   [ ] Yes   [ ] No

   _____ (24)

6.   If yes, when did you want to eat? (Tick any box which applies).

                                        Early labour [ ]   _____ (25)
                                      Middle labour [ ]   _____ (26)
                                      Late labour [ ]

   _____ (27)

7.   Were you allowed to eat within reason what you wanted?   [ ] Yes   [ ] No   _____ (28)

8.   If no, what was the reason? _____

   _____

9.   The following people may have been with you <u>during your labour</u>. Please say whether or not
      they were there and whether you were pleased that they were there. Please tick any box
      which applies in each row.

	Present during labour	I was pleased they were there	
Husband/partner	[ ]	[ ]	_____ (29-30)
Children	[ ]	[ ]	_____ (31-32)
Mother	[ ]	[ ]	_____ (33-34)
Known midwife	[ ]	[ ]	_____ (35-36)
Other midwife	[ ]	[ ]	_____ (37-38)
Student midwife	[ ]	[ ]	_____ (39-40)
GP	[ ]	[ ]	_____ (41-42)
Obstetrician	[ ]	[ ]	_____ (43-44)
Anaesthetist	[ ]	[ ]	_____ (45-46)
Paediatrician (baby's doctor)	[ ]	[ ]	_____ (47-48)
Student doctor	[ ]	[ ]	_____ (49-50)
Student nurse	[ ]	[ ]	_____ (51-52)
Friends	[ ]	[ ]	_____ (53-54)
Others	[ ]	[ ]	_____ (55-56)

   _____ (57)

   (specify) _____

5

260

BLUE QUESTIONNAIRE

10. The following people may have been with you <u>at the birth of your baby</u>. Please say whether or not they were there and whether you were pleased that they were there. Please tick any box which applies in each row.

	Present at the birth	I was pleased they were there
Husband/partner		
Children		
Mother		
Known midwife		
Other midwife		
Student midwife		
GP		
Obstetrician		
Anaesthetist		
Paediatrician (baby's doctor)		
Student doctor		
Student nurse		
Friends		
Others		

(specify) _____

_____ (1-3)
_____ (4-7)
__03___ (8-9)

_____ (10-11)
_____ (12-13)
_____ (14-15)
_____ (16-17)
_____ (18-19)
_____ (20-21)
_____ (22-23)
_____ (24-25)
_____ (26-27)
_____ (28-29)
_____ (30-31)
_____ (32-33)
_____ (34-35)
_____ (36-37)
_____ (38)

11. What did you use to help relieve the pain of labour and what did you find helpful? (Please tick any box which applies in each row).

	Used	Helpful
None		
Relaxation/breathing exercises		
Massage		
Warm water		
TENS		
Acupuncture		
Homeopathy		
Aromatherapy		
Injection eg. Pethidine		
Entonox (gas & oxygen)		
Epidural		
Spinal		
General anaesthetic		
Other		

(specify) _____

_____ (39-40)
_____ (41-42)
_____ (43-44)
_____ (45-46)
_____ (47-48)
_____ (49-50)
_____ (51-52)
_____ (53-54)
_____ (55-56)
_____ (57-58)
_____ (59-60)
_____ (61-62)
_____ (63-64)
_____ (65-66)
_____ (67)

D. AFTER THE BIRTH OF YOUR BABY

_____ (1-3)
_____ (4-7)
__04___ (8-9)

1. Did you experience any of the following problems in the first 48 hours after the birth of the baby? (Tick any that apply).

Tiredness		Headache	
Backache		Painful stitches	
Constipation		Piles	
Breast problems		Tearfulness	
Abnormal vaginal bleeding		Urine infection	
Leaking urine		High blood pressure	
Other			

(Specify) _____

_____ (10-11)
_____ (12-13)
_____ (14-15)
_____ (16-17)
_____ (18-19)
_____ (20-21)
_____ (22)

_____ (23)

6

261

2. How are you feeding your baby? (Please tick one box).

    Breast milk only
    Breast & bottle milk
    Bottle milk only
    _____ (24)

3. Is this how you had planned to feed your baby?   Yes ☐   No ☐
    _____ (25)

4. When you fed your baby for the first time, how did the baby respond? (Tick any that apply)

    Fed well   Irritable   _____ (26-27)
    Not interested   Was sick   _____ (28-29)
    Sleepy   Other   _____ (30-31)
                                             _____ (32)
                          (specify) _____

5. Were you happy about your decision to have a hospital birth? (Tick one box only)

    1. Very happy
    2. Moderately happy
    3. Not very happy
    4. Rather unhappy
    _____ (33)

6. What did you like __most__ about having your baby in hospital?

    _____
    _____ (34)
    _____

7. What did you like __least__ about having your baby in hospital?

    _____
    _____ (35)
    _____

8. How do you feel about the care you received from the midwives at birth? (Tick one box).

    1. Very satisfied
    2. Satisfied
    3. Dissatisfied
    4. Very dissatisfied
    5. Don't know
    _____ (36)

9. How do you feel about the care you received from the doctors at birth? (Tick one box).

    1. Very satisfied
    2. Satisfied
    3. Dissatisfied
    4. Very dissatisfied
    5. Don't know
    6. Not applicable
    _____ (37)

10. If you have another baby, where would you choose to give birth? (Tick one box).

    1. Same place as this time
    2. Home rather than hospital
    3. GP unit
    4. Other hospital
    5. Other
        (specify) _____
    _____ (38)
    _____ (39)

7

262

BLUE QUESTIONNAIRE

11. How many days are you planning to stay/did you stay in hospital? [|] Number

_____ (40-41)

12. Do you feel your stay in hospital was : (Tick one box only)

_____ (42)

    1. Too short   [   ]   2. Too long   [   ]
    3. Just right   [   ]   4. Don't know

Thank you very much for completing this form. The following space has been left blank for any other comments you or your husband/partner would like to make.

E. **COMMENTS**

1. Your comments

_____ (43)

2. Your partner's comments

_____ (44)

8

APPENDIX IV

NATIONAL BIRTHDAY TRUST

1994 ENQUIRY INTO HOME BIRTHS

To the midwife caring for the woman who planned to give birth in hospital.

Dear Colleague,

BACKGROUND TO THE SURVEY

Discussions continue about the wishes of women to deliver where they choose and the relative safety of home and hospital birth (Changing Childbirth 1993); there are still few real facts about the different experiences in the two places. The National Birthday Trust is conducting a National Survey to collect data from both consumers and professionals to learn more about home births.

The main aim of the study is to collect information on every birth which, at 37 weeks gestation, is planned at home. In order to compare that information with a planned hospital birth, a woman with a background similar to the home birth mother needs to be identified.

YOUR INVOLVEMENT IN THE STUDY

I ask for your help with the relevant questionnaires and also to distribute forms to the appropriate women who have agreed to participate. You will note that a NBT Home Births Study label has been attached to the notes of women who have been entered into the survey. The study is entirely voluntary but I hope that you and the women will agree to take part because the greater the response, the more valid the findings.

Once the baby has been born, please complete a yellow questionnaire and give it to the Supervisor of Midwives who is co-ordinating the collection of forms in your district. Could you also give a blue questionnaire to the woman, ask her to complete it within the first 48 hours of the postnatal period if possible and explain to her that a pre-paid envelope is enclosed so she can post it directly to me.

If the baby is stillborn or dies soon after birth, I would be grateful if you would still complete your form. In previous studies, women whose baby died have indicated that they still want to relate their experiences; if you feel that it is appropriate, contact your Supervisor of Midwives who will give you the relevant questionnaire for the woman to complete.

CONFIDENTIALITY

All the information you give is fully confidential. When the forms are returned to the survey office, all personal and geographical details will be replaced with a survey code and from then on the questionnaires will have a number only.

I appreciate the time this consumes and I thank you for your committment to this national enquiry.

Ann Wraight

1

YELLOW QUESTIONNAIRE

Six weeks after the delivery, a random sample of women will be sent a second short questionnaire so that any shift in attitudes and any problems experienced can be identified in both groups.

The following information is therefore required to enable the research team to contact the woman at home.

When this form reaches the survey office, this page will be detached so that the questionnaire is rendered anonymous and cannot be traced to individuals.

Woman's Name _____

Woman's Address _____

_____

postcode _____

Health Authority/Board/Trust _____

Address where baby was born :
_____
_____

postcode _____

FOR OFFICE
USE ONLY

_____

_____

2

How to fill in this questionnaire:

Most questions can be answered by ticking the box or boxes which apply to you. Please ignore the numbers in or beside the boxes, they are to help me analyse the answers.

Sometimes I would like you to fill in a number in the box(es), and in a few cases I would like you to write in your answer in your own words.

Go from one question to the next unless the box you have ticked tells you otherwise. In this way you will miss out the questions which do not apply to you.

Please feel free to write in extra comments if you would like to give me more information.

Ann Wraight.

A.	DESCRIPTIVE DATA ABOUT THE WOMAN

1.   PAST PREGNANCIES (24 weeks gestation and above):

FOR OFFICE USE ONLY

Year	Site of delivery e.g. home/ hospital	Method of delivery	Gestation	Outcome live/ stillbirth	Birthweight (gm)

_____ (1-3)
_____ (4-7)
___01___ (8-9)

_____ (10-16)

_____ (17-23)

_____ (24-30)

_____ (31-37)

_____ (38-44)

PRESENT PREGNANCY :

2.   At what stage of gestation did the booking take place?   Weeks [|]   _____ (45-46)

3.   Did you attend the woman during her pregnancy?   Yes [ ]   No [ ]   _____ (47)

4.   If yes, how many antenatal visits were done by you?   Number [|]   _____ (48-49)

5.   Was an ultrasound scan (not Doppler) performed in pregnancy?   Yes [ ]   No [ ]   _____ (50)

6.   Was antenatal CTG performed?   Yes [ ]   No [ ]   _____ (51)

7.   Were any other special tests/investigations performed? e.g. amniocentesis, Doppler   Yes [ ]   No [ ]   _____ (52)

8.   If yes, please specify _____   _____ (53)
_____ (54)
_____ (55)

_____

9.   Did any of the following complications occur in pregnancy? (Tick any that apply).

_____ (56-57)
_____ (58-59)
_____ (60-61)
_____ (62-63)
_____ (64)

Hypertensive disease	[ ]	Cardiac disease	[ ]
Diabetes	[ ]	Antepartum haemorrhage	[ ]
Mental illness	[ ]	Intrauterine growth retardation	[ ]
Pre-eclampsia/PIH	[ ]	Other	[ ]

(specify) _____

3

YELLOW QUESTIONNAIRE

10. PLACE OF BIRTH (Tick one box only in each column) :

	Intended place of birth	Actual place of birth
1. Home		
2. GP unit		
3. Midwife led care		
4. GP bed		
5. Consultant bed		
6. Ambulance		_____ (65-66)
7. Other		_____ (67)

(specify) _____

11. PROFESSIONAL SUPPORT
Please specify in each column the number of people who attended the woman during pregnancy, labour and delivery.

_____ (1-3)
_____ (4-7)
__02__ (8-9)

	Pregnancy (Specify no.)	Labour (Specify no.)	Delivery (Specify no.)	
Known midwife -				
community				_____ (10-13)
hospital				_____ (14-17)
independent				_____ (18-21)
Other midwife				_____ (22-25)
Own GP				_____ (26-29)
Other GP				_____ (30-33)
SHO				_____ (34-37)
Registrar/Senior Reg.				_____ (38-41)
Consultant				_____ (42-45)
Other				_____ (46-49)
				_____ (50)

(specify) _____

....

B. LABOUR

1. Was the labour induced?   Yes [___]   No [___]

_____ (51)

2. When did each stage begin? (Please give date and time, use 24 hour clock).

_____ (1-3)
_____ (4-7)
__03__ (8-9)

	Date	Time
1. 1st stage	__/__/__	
2. 2nd stage	__/__/__	
3. 3rd stage	__/__/__	

3. When did the 3rd stage end? (Please give date and time)

_____ (10-19)
_____ (20-29)
_____ (30-39)

Date __/__/__   Time [_____]

4. When did you arrive at the house/take over her care in labour? (Please give date and time)

_____ (40-49)

Date __/__/__   Time [_____]

_____ (50-59)

5. Had the woman completed a written plan of her wishes for labour?   Yes [___]   No [___]

_____ (60)

6. If yes, was it followed?   Yes [___]   No [___]

_____ (61)

7. If no, please specify the main reason _____

_____ (62)

4

8. Pain relief used (Tick any that apply) :

None	☐	Relaxation/breathing exercises	☐
Entonox		TENS	
Meptazinol		Acupuncture	
Pethidine		Homeopathy	
Diamorphine/Morphine		Aromatherapy	
Epidural		Massage	
Spinal		Warm water	
General Anaesthetic	☐	Other	☐

(specify) _____

(63-64)
(65-66)
(67-68)
(69-70)
(71-72)
(73-74)
(75-76)
(77-78)
(79)

(80)

9. Were the forewaters ruptured artificially?   Yes ☐   No ☐

(1-3)
(4-7)
04 (8-9)

10. If yes, what was the cervical dilatation?   ☐☐ cm

(10-11)

11. What position was adopted for delivery (Tick one box only).

1. Propped up in bed	☐	2. Lithotomy	☐	
3. Supine with lateral tilt		4. All fours		
5. Sitting		6. Standing		
7. Birth chair		8. Lateral		
9. Supine		10. Squatting	☐	
11. Other	☐			

(specify)_____

(12-13)

(14)

12. Did the birth take place in water?   Yes ☐   No ☐

(15)

13. Method of delivery (Tick one box only).

Spontaneous -		Assisted -	
1. occipito anterior	☐	5. forceps	☐
2. occipito posterior		6. vacuum extraction	
3. breech		7. Caesarean Section	
4. face	☐	8. Other	☐

(specify) _____

(16)

(17)

5

YELLOW QUESTIONNAIRE

14. Personnel present at time of birth.

	Who delivered the baby? (Tick one box)	Who was the lead professional at the delivery? (Tick one box)	Who else (i.e. staff) were present at the delivery? (Specify the number present in each relevant box)	
E grade midwife				_____ (18-20)
F grade midwife				_____ (21-23)
G grade midwife				_____ (24-26)
H grade midwife				_____ (27-29)
I grade midwife				_____ (30-32)
Independent midwife				_____ (33-35)
Student midwife				_____ (36-38)
GP				_____ (39-41)
Medical student				_____ (42-44)
SHO				_____ (45-47)
Registrar				_____ (48-50)
Senior registrar				_____ (51-53)
Consultant				_____ (54-56)
Anaesthetist				_____ (57-59)
Paediatrician				_____ (60-62)
Ambulance Officer				_____ (63-65)
Other				_____ (66-68)

(specify) _____   _____ (69)

15. Management of 3rd stage. (Tick any that apply) :

Physiological		_____ (70)
Controlled cord traction		_____ (71)
Manual removal of placenta		_____ (72)
Syntometrine/Ergometrine		_____ (73)
Syntocinon		_____ (74)
Other		_____ (75)
		_____ (76)

(specify) _____

    _____ (1-3)

16. Estimated blood loss   [| | |]   ml   _____ (4-7)

    __05__ (8-9)

17. Perineal damage. (Tick any that apply) :

None		_____ (10-13)
1st degree tear		
2nd degree tear		_____ (14)
3rd degree tear		_____ (15)
Episiotomy		_____ (16)
Vaginal tear		_____ (17)
Cervical tear		_____ (18)
		_____ (19)
		_____ (20)

18. Who repaired the tear/episiotomy? (Tick one box only) :

1. Midwife who delivered baby   2. GP
3. Other midwife   4. SHO
5. Registrar   6. Consultant   _____ (21)
7. Other

(specify) _____   _____ (22)

6

269

19. What suture material was used? (Tick any that apply) :

Catgut ☐   Dexon ☐
Silk ☐   Dexon/vicryl ☐
Other ☐

_____ (23-24)
_____ (25-26)
(specify) _____
_____ (27)

20. When did the repair take place? (Please give date and time)
_____ (28)

Date   __/__/__   Time ☐☐☐☐☐
_____ (29-38)

21. Did any complications occur in labour which have not already been mentioned?
_____ (39)

Yes ☐   No ☐
_____ (40)
_____ (41)
22. If yes, please specify _____
_____ (42)

....

C.   BABY

1. What was the outcome? (Tick one box only)

Livebirth ☐   Stillbirth ☐   Neonatal Death ☐
_____ (43)

2. What was the gestation? ☐☐ weeks
_____ (44-45)

3. What was the birthweight? ☐☐☐☐ gm
_____ (46-49)

4. What were the Apgar scores?   1 minute ☐☐   5 minutes ☐☐
_____ (50-53)

5. Was the baby resuscitated?   Yes ☐   No ☐
_____ (54)

6. If yes, what resuscitation was required? (Tick any that apply).

Aspiration ☐
Bag and mask ☐
Intubation ☐
_____ (55)
_____ (56)
_____ (57)

7. If yes, who resuscitated the baby? (Tick any that apply).

Midwife ☐   GP ☐
Paediatrician ☐   Obstetrician ☐
Anaesthetist ☐   Other ☐
_____ (58-59)
_____ (60-61)
_____ (62-63)

(specify) _____
_____ (64)

8. Were there any birth injuries?   Yes ☐   No ☐
_____ (65)

9. If yes, please specify _____
_____ (66)
_____ (67)
10. Were there any congenital abnormalities? Yes ☐   No ☐
_____ (68)

11. If yes, please specify _____
_____ (69)

12. Did the baby require specialist care? Yes ☐   No ☐
_____ (70-71)
_____ (72-73)
_____ (74-75)

_____ (76)

7

YELLOW QUESTIONNAIRE

13.   If yes, where was the baby transferred?   (Tick one box only)

     1. Neonatal unit   ☐   2. Surgical unit   ☐
     3. Maternity unit   ☐   4. Other   ☐

                            (specify) _____

14.   When was the baby transferred? (Please give date and time)

         Date   __/__/__   Time   ☐☐☐☐

15.   Was the admission   1.Planned   ☐   2.Emergency   ☐

16.   What were the reasons for transfer? _____

_____

Thank you very much for completing this form. The remainder of this page has been left blank for any other comments you would like to make.

_____	(1-3)
_____	(4-7)
__06__	(8-9)
_____	(10)
_____	(11)
,	
_____	(12-21)
_____	(22)
_____	(23)
_____	(24)
_____	(25)

8

APPENDIX V

THE NATIONAL BIRTHDAY TRUST

1994 ENQUIRY INTO HOME BIRTHS

You will remember that a few weeks ago, when your baby was born, your midwife gave you a questionnaire to complete to give us details of your labour and delivery.Thank you very much for completing that. The information I have received is very helpful and I am in the process of the first analysis.

I now ask you to help me with this second (and last) questionnaire so I can compare your views now with those you had soon after the birth of your baby. The answers you give will be <u>entirely confidential</u>. Your name does not appear on the questionnaire and no mention about the results of individual women will be made available. Your midwife does not participate in this part of the survey and will know nothing of your answers. The study will provide information to help improve the care given to women by the health services throughout the UK.

I am indebted to you for your help. Please post the form back as soon as possible in the pre-paid envelope enclosed.

Thank you again for taking part in this study.

Ann Wraight
Midwife Co-ordinator
The National Birthday Trust
Department of Obstetrics and Gynaecology
St George's Hospital
Cranmer Terrace
London SW17 0RE

1

CREAM QUESTIONNAIRE

CONFIDENTIAL

How to fill in this questionnaire :

Most questions can be answered by ticking the box or boxes which apply to you. Please ignore numbers in or beside the boxes. They are to help me analyse the answers.

Sometimes I would like you to fill in a number in the boxes, and in a few cases I would like you to write in your answer in your own words.

Go from one question to the next unless the box you have ticked tells you otherwise. In this way you will miss out questions which do not apply to you.

Please feel free to write in extra comments if you would like to give me more information.

Ann Wraight

FOR OFFICE
USE ONLY

_____ (1-3)
_____ (4-7)
__01__ (8-9)

PLACE OF BIRTH

1. How old is your baby? Enter number of weeks.   [|]   _____ (10-11)

2. Do you feel you made the right choice about where you had your baby?

   Yes [ ]   No [ ]   Don't know [ ]   _____ (12)

3. What makes you feel like this?
   _____
   _____   _____ (13)

4. If you have another baby, where would you choose to give birth? (Tick one box only)

   1. Home
   2. GP unit
   3. Hospital   _____ (14)

5. If hospital which type of care would you prefer? (Tick one box only)

   1. Midwife led care
   2. Birth room
   3. DOMINO
   4. GP led care
   5. Consultant led care
   6. Other   _____ (15)

      (specify) _____   _____ (16)

FEELINGS ABOUT THE BIRTH :

6. On the whole did you enjoy the birth of your baby?

   Yes [ ]   No [ ]   Don't know [ ]   _____ (17)

7. How much in control of the labour did you feel? (Tick one box only).

   1. Completely in control
   2. Quite in control
   3. Not very in control
   4. Not at all in control
   5. Don't know   _____ (18)

2

273

8. How much pain would you say you felt during the labour? (Tick one box only).

   1. No pain at all
   2. Very little pain
   3. Some pain
   4. A great deal of pain
   5. Don't know

   _____ (19)

9. Have you had any of the following health problems <u>at home</u> since you have had your baby? (Please tick each problem you have had and each one which was treated).

	Problem	Problem treated by doctor	
Tiredness			
Headache			_____ (20-21)
Backache			_____ (22-23)
Painful stitches			_____ (24-25)
Constipation			_____ (26-27)
Piles			_____ (28-29)
Breast problems			_____ (30-31)
Tearfulness or depression			_____ (32-33)
Abnormal bleeding from vagina			_____ (34-35)
Urine infection			_____ (36-37)
Leaking urine			_____ (38-39)
High blood pressure			_____ (40-41)
Other			_____ (42-43)
			_____ (44-45)

   (specify) _____ _____ (46)

10. Did you have to be admitted to hospital after the birth of your baby?   Yes [ ]   No [ ]   _____ (47)

11. If yes, please give reasons : _____   _____ (48)

   _____   _____ (49)

12. Has your baby been admitted to hospital since birth?   Yes [ ]   No [ ]   _____ (50)

   _____ (51)

13. If yes, please give reasons : _____   _____ (52)

14. Since <u>the birth of your baby</u>, how have you felt in yourself? (Tick one box only).

   1. Very happy
   2. Happy
   3. Quite depressed
   4. Very depressed
   5. Don't know

   _____ (53)

15. How confident do you feel as a mother? (Tick one box only).

   1. Very confident about everything
   2. Confident about most things
   3. Not very confident
   4. Not at all confident
   5. Don't know

   _____ (54)

3

CREAM QUESTIONNAIRE

16. How are you feeding your baby now? (Tick one box only).

1. Breast milk only
2. Bottle milk only
3. Both breast and bottle milks
4. Other

_____ (55)

(specify) _____

_____ (56)

....

THE PROVISION OF MATERNITY SERVICES

Do you have any comments on the way care is provided for pregnant women and new mothers in the UK? Please use this last section to write any comments you think would be helpful.

16. YOUR COMMENTS :

_____ (57)

17. YOUR HUSBAND'S/PARTNER'S COMMENTS :

_____ (58)

Thank you once again for the help you have given us in this study.

4

APPENDIX VI

ORANGE QUESTIONNAIRE

FOR OFFICE
USE ONLY

HOME BIRTHS - NOT REGISTERED IN THIS STUDY

To the Supervisor of Midwives filling out this questionnaire :

Please complete one form for every birth which takes place in the home which was not planned to be there. This includes unbooked pregnancies, those which had been booked for hospital or GP unit delivery and also those who all along had intended to give birth at home but had not booked for a home birth by 37 weeks gestation.

_____ (1-3)
_____ (4-7)

Ann Wraight

___01___ (8-9)

1. Was this a booked pregnancy? (Tick one box only)

    1. Yes, at this hospital
    2. Yes, at another hospital
    3. Yes, at home after 37 weeks
    4. No, not booked anywhere

    _____ (10)

2. If the pregnancy was not booked, what was the main reason? _____

    _____ (11)

3. Was the outcome? (Tick one box only)

    1. Livebirth [   ]   2. Stillbirth [   ]   3. Neonatal death [   ]

4. What was the gestational age of the baby?   [|] Weeks

    _____ (12)

5. What was the woman's parity? (Tick one box only)

    1. 0 [   ]   2. 1-4 [   ]   3. >4 [   ]

    _____ (13-14)

    _____ (15)

6. What was the **main** reason for the unplanned or unbooked home birth? (Tick one box only).

    1. Preterm labour   [   ]   2. Concealed pregnancy   [   ]
    3. No available transport   [   ]   4. Quick labour   [   ]
    5. She refused hospital delivery [ ]   6. Not encouraged by doctor [   ]
    7. Not encouraged by midwife [   ]   8. Not encouraged by family [   ]
    8. Other   [   ]

    _____ (16)

    _____ (17)

        (specify)_____

7. Who delivered the baby and who else was present at the birth?

	Who delivered the baby? (Tick box)	Who else was present? (specify actual number)	
No assistant	[ ]	[ ]	(18-19)
Husband/partner	[ ]	[ ]	(20-21)
Neighbour	[ ]	[ ]	(22-23)
Family member	[ ]	[ ]	(24-25)
Friend	[ ]	[ ]	(26-27)
Ambulance officer	[ ]	[ ]	(28-29)
Midwife	[ ]	[ ]	(30-31)
GP	[ ]	[ ]	(32-33)
Hospital doctor	[ ]	[ ]	(34-35)
Don't know	[ ]	[ ]	(36-37)
Other	[ ]	[ ]	(38-39)
			(40)

        (specify) _____

* NB PLEASE COMPLETE THE REVERSE SIDE OF THIS FORM

ORANGE QUESTIONNAIRE

8. Was there any transfer to hospital? (Tick one box only).

1. Yes, mother and baby
2. No, neither mother nor baby
3. Yes, mother only
4. Yes, baby only

_____ (41)

9. If yes to 8, which method of transport was used? (Tick one box only)

_____ (42)

1. Obstetric flying squad
2. Neonatal flying squad
3. Ambulance with paramedics
4. Ambulance with midwife
5. Ambulance with midwife and paramedics
6. Car
7. Helicopter/plane
8. Other

_____ (43)

(specify) _____

10. If yes to 8, which of the following methods of treatment took place (Tick all relevant boxes)

a) **Mother**
Manual removal of placenta   Blood transfusion
Repair of laceration   Other

(specify)_____

_____ (﹨)
_____ (46-47)
_____ (48)

b) **Baby**
Incubator care   Respiratory support
Neonatal surgery   Other

(specify)_____

_____ (49-50)
_____ (51-52)
_____ (53)

11. Please add any comments which you feel are important :

_____ (5 ﹨)

Name of supervisor : _____   Date : ___/___/___

Address : _____

_____

_____

postcode _____

Thank you very much for completing this form. Please return it to me in the enclosed pre-paid envelope.

Ann Wraight, The National Birthday Trust
Department of Obstetrics and Gynaecology, St George's Hospital Medical School
Cranmer Terrace, London SW17 ORE

Glossary

Accoucheur An historical name for an obstetrician.

Acupuncture Stimulation by needle insertion into the skin at specific points of the body to alleviate pain.

Amniocentesis The removal of a small amount of amniotic fluid for laboratory analysis usually of the chromosomes in the nuclei of the fetal cells suspended in the fluid. Commonly performed at about 16 weeks of pregnancy although some hospitals do it earlier.

Anaesthetist Doctor who specializes in the administration of anaesthetics and drugs that relieve pain.

Antepartum haemorrhage Bleeding from the genital tract between the 24th week of pregnancy and labour.

Apgar score A scoring index which helps to assess the condition of a baby at birth.

Aromatherapy Use of massage and fragrant oils to relieve the pain of labour.

Aspiration pneumonitis Inflammation of the lungs produced by the inhalation of vomit containing acid stomach contents.

Asphyxia Severe reduction in oxygen levels following poor transfer across the placenta to the fetus or later from the inability of the newborn baby to breathe spontaneously.

Augmentation Acceleration of labour following a spontaneous onset to increase the efficiency of uterine contractions when progress is slow.

Bach's Rescue Remedy Inexpensive homeopathic flower remedy which is used in labour to relieve anxiety. A few drops are added to a small amount of water or dropped straight on to the tongue.

Bag and mask resuscitation Artificial respiration of the baby using a bag and close-fitting face mask to get air or oxygen into the lungs under pressure.

Birth plan A written plan of a woman's preferences for her care to discuss with her professionals during the antenatal period well before labour.

Birthroom A room, in or close to a maternity unit, which is furnished in a comfortable, attractive and home-like fashion and capable of being transformed into an efficient delivery area.

Breech Delivery in which baby's buttocks present first.

Caesarean section An operation performed to deliver the baby through an incision in the abdominal wall and the uterus so bypassing the vaginal route.

Caput succedaneum Localized swelling on the baby's scalp formed during labour as a result of circular pressure of the cervix or a vacuum cap.

Cardiotocograph (CTG) The monitoring and recording of the fetal heartbeat and uterine contractions.

Cardiac Relating to the heart.

Cephalhaematoma Swelling on baby's scalp caused by bleeding under the skin.

Cephalic Relating to the head.

Cervix Neck of the uterus or womb.

Cleft palate A fissure in the palate when the two sides fail to fuse during the development stage of the fetus.

Compound presentation When more than one part of the fetus presents in the labour at the same time, e.g. a head and a hand together.

Consultant Specialist doctor who is ultimately responsible for the management of women admitted to hospital under his care. He directs the policies of the medical teams.

Contractions Rhythmic tightenings of the muscles in the uterus to expel the fetus.

Controlled cord traction Active management of the third stage of labour when traction is applied on the cord with counter pressure applied to the contracted uterus through the wall of the abdomen.

Cord prolapse When the membranes rupture, the cord is found to be lying in front of the presenting part in the cervical canal or vagina.

Diabetes Disease caused by deficient secretion of insulin allowing blood sugars to rise. Maternal diabetes can affect the fetus.

Diamorphine Strong, long-lasting analgesic occasionally given to relieve the pain of labour.

DOMINO A plan of care when the mother gives birth in a maternity unit, cared for by the community midwife who has looked after her antenatally. They return home usually within hours of birth. Abbreviation for DOMiciliary IN/Out.

Doppler ultrasound A technique using ultrasound to monitor the flow of a moving column of fluid such as blood flow through uterine arteries or the vessels of the umbilical cord.

Eclampsia A serious complication of pregnancy characterized by fits and accompanied by severe high blood pressure, fluid retention and protein in the urine.

Entonox A mixture of 50% nitrous oxide and 50% oxygen, used as an analgesic which is breathed in.

Epidural A local anaesthetic injected outside the spinal sac so numbing the nerve roots as they arrive at the spinal cord. This leads to a temporary loss of sensation in the lower part of the body. It is used in labour to abolish the pain of uterine contractions, or as an alternative to general anaesthetic during Caesarean section.

Episiotomy A surgical procedure in which an incision is made in the perineum to enlarge the vaginal opening if necessary for the birth of the baby.

Ergometrine A drug given to help the uterus contract in the prevention or treatment of postpartum haemorrhage.

Face presentation A presentation of the baby in labour in which the head of the baby is extended so that the face presents lowest in the pelvis and delivers first.

Fetal distress A compromised condition of the fetus usually caused by lack of oxygen. It is sometimes characterized by a markedly abnormal rate or rhythm of the heart.

Fetus Term given to the unborn baby after the 8th week of pregnancy.

Forceps delivery Method of assisting the delivery of the baby in the second stage of labour by application of suitable curved metal spoon-like blades on each side of the baby's head.

General anaesthetic Agents given to a patient to bring about complete loss of consciousness and consequent unawareness of any painful stimuli. It is commonly used for surgical operations.

General practitioners Family doctors with total overall care of their patients. They are the primary health practitioners but may have extra experience and qualifications in different specialities, e.g. obstetrics.

Gestation Pregnancy.

Gravidity The number of times a woman has been pregnant.

Homeopathy Medicines used in very small doses. Some find this helpful to relieve the pain of labour.

Hydrocoele An accumulation of fluid around the testicles. In the newborn it is often caused by failure of the canal between the scrotum and peritoneal cavity to close during fetal development.

Index pregnancy The present or current pregnancy in a study.

Induction Procedure to start labour artificially where prolongation of the pregnancy would put the health of mother or fetus at risk.

Inferior vena cava The large vein that carries deoxygenated blood back to the heart from the lower parts of the body.

Intubation Insertion of a semi-rigid tube through the mouth or nose to ensure the airway to the lungs stays open when the patient is unconscious.

Intrauterine growth retardation (IUGR)   Delay in fetal growth resulting in the baby being small for gestational age.

Intravenous (i.v.)   Within a vein.

Labour   The process of delivery, which takes place in three stages: first – opening of the neck of the uterus (cervix); second – birth of the baby; third – expulsion of the afterbirth (placenta).

Larynx   The voice box, a part of the air passage connecting pharynx with trachea.

Lithotomy   A position where the woman lies supine with the legs supported so that the hips and knees are flexed and the thighs are apart.

Local Supervising Authority   The authority designated to undertake the statutory supervision of midwives according to the rules of the United Kingdom Central Council (UKCC).

Low birth weight   A weight of 2500 g or less at birth.

Malpresentation   Any presentation of the fetus other than the vertex, e.g. breech, brow.

Manual removal of placenta   The introduction of a doctor's hand into the uterus in order to remove a placenta which has been retained.

Massage   Stroking, rubbing, or kneading of neck, trunk and limb muscles to assist relaxation and so help relieve the pain of labour.

Midwife   One who specializes in the care of women during pregnancy, childbirth and the puerperium. She or he may practise independently or as an employee within a hospital or community. The post held is graded from E to I (E being the most junior) according to the responsibilities.

Meptazinol (Meptid)   Short-term drug used to relieve the pain of labour.

Multigravida   A woman who has been pregnant more than once.

Neonatal death   Death of a baby within 28 days of birth. If such a death occurs in the first 7 days, it is categorized as an early neonatal death; such early neonatal deaths are grouped with stillbirths to derive the perinatal mortality rate.

Neonatal Narcan   Drug given to baby to counteract respiratory depression caused by the mother having opioids or other respiratory depressant in labour.

Neonatal unit   A special ward or intensive care nursery which provides continuous skilled supervision of sick newborn babies.

Obstetric flying squad   A team of obstetric and midwifery personnel which used to be available to provide emergency treatment to the mother away from the main obstetrical hospital of a district.

Obstetrician   A doctor who specializes in the care of pregnant women and their babies in pregnancy, at their deliveries and in the postnatal period.

Occipito anterior (OA)   Position when the back of the baby's head is to the front of the mother's pelvis as the head descends through the birth canal. This is a favourable position for delivery.

Occipito posterior (OP)   Position when the back of the baby's head is towards the back of the mother's pelvis. This is an unfavourable position for delivery.

Occipito transverse (OT)   Position when the back of the baby's head lies on either side of the mother's pelvis. This is usually transient occurring in pregnancy and early labour. With descent, most babies are rotated to OA or less commonly to OP.

Opiate   A drug containing opium given to relieve pain.

Oxytocic agent   One of the drugs which causes the smooth muscle of the uterus to contract.

Paediatric flying squad   A team of paediatricians and neonatal nurses available to provide emergency treatment to the newborn baby away from the hospital housing a special care baby unit.

Paediatrician   A doctor specializing in the care of infants and children. Some paediatricians specialize in caring for the newborn – neonatologists.

Palsy   The loss of muscle function.

Paramedic   Ambulance personnel with special training in emergency medical procedures.

Parity   The number of times a woman has given birth to a baby.

Perinatal mortality rate   The number of stillbirths and early neonatal deaths per 1000 live births.

Perineal tear   Tear sustained in the area between the vagina and anus. A first-degree tear involves the skin only; a second-degree tear involves the skin and muscle layers; a third-degree tear involves skin, muscle and extends into the anal sphincter.

Pethidine   A moderately strong analgesic used to relieve the pain of labour.

Placenta   The interchange organ through which the fetus obtains oxygen and nutrients and excretes carbon dioxide and other waste products. The placenta ceases to act as a transfer station once the baby has been born and it is expelled as the afterbirth.

Postpartum haemorrhage   Excessive bleeding (more than 500 ml) after the birth of the baby.

Pre-eclampsia   An abnormal condition of pregnancy characterized by the onset of raised blood pressure accompanied by protein in the urine and sometimes water retention leading to puffiness of the tissues.

Primigravida   A woman who is pregnant for the first time.

Primiparous   A woman having her first baby.

Prolonged labour   Labour which extends beyond the usual time span when the uterus is contracting efficiently, e.g. over 18 h of full uterine contractions in a primigravida and 12 h in a multigravida.

Registrar   A doctor who has practised as a Senior House Officer for 2 years and is now continuing training in a chosen specialty. During this training an obstetric registrar will obtain a higher diploma as a Member of the Royal College of Obstetricians and Gynaecologists.

Relaxation exercises   Exercises practised in pregnancy and performed in labour aimed to reduce tension with the contractions during labour.

Senior house officer   A doctor who has completed a year of general medical and surgical training after qualification and has now joined a specialty, e.g. obstetrics. Commonly doctors spend 2 years at this level during which they obtained a Diploma of the RCOG.

Senior registrar   Doctors who have been promoted from registrar level where they have worked for 3 or 4 years. Most become consultants in 3–4 years.

Shared care   A system of care carried out by a midwife and a general practitioner or an obstetrician.

Shoulder dystocia   An emergency occurring during labour when the baby's shoulders fail to turn spontaneously after the birth of the head and become jammed in the pelvis so preventing further descent.

Sonicaid   Ultrasound apparatus used to detect the fetal heart rate.

Spinal anaesthetic   Injection of an analgesic or anaesthetic drug into the fluid bathing the spinal cord. This differs from an epidural anaesthetic for it numbs sensation by blocking at a higher level of the nervous system.

Stillbirth   A baby born dead after the 24th week of pregnancy.

Supervisor of Midwives   A senior midwife appointed by the Local Supervising Authority to exercise supervision over all hospital or community midwives in her locality. She supervises both NHS and independent midwives.

Syntocinon   A synthetic oxytocin which acts in the same way as pitocin but is a purer preparation.

Syntometrine   An oxytocic combination of drugs (syntocinon and ergometrine) commonly administered to the mother to help the delivery of the placenta and lessen blood loss.

Talipes   Congenital deformity of the foot and ankle.

TENS (transcutaneous electrical nerve stimulation)   A method of pain relief in labour. Electrodes are placed on the skin to produce a pulsed electrical current which interrupts pain transmission and may stimulate the production of endogenous opiates.

Trachea   Passage which conveys air from the throat to the lungs.

Triple test   A test performed in pregnancy to measure three hormones in the blood which show the woman a degree of risk of carrying a Down's syndrome baby. It is usually performed at about 16 weeks of pregnancy.

Ultrasound   The use of pulsed high-frequency sound to produce images of the fetus, placenta and uterus during pregnancy.

Uterus   A hollow muscle sac in which the fetus grows for the length of pregnancy. The womb.

Vacuum extraction   A method of delivering the baby by applying a suction cup to the baby's head. The scalp is then drawn gently into the cap by the use of the vacuum and the baby is guided through the birth canal with the assistance of traction.

Vagina   The canal which runs from the cervix of the uterus to the exterior at the vulva.

Index